PHYSICAL FITNESS ASTRONAUT TRAINING MANUAL

A. EUGENE COLEMAN

FOR
THE NATIONAL AERONAUTICS
SPACE ADMINISTRATION

Fredonia Books
Amsterdam, The Netherlands

Physical Fitness Astronaut Training Manual

by
A. Eugene Coleman

For
The National Aeronautics Space Administration

ISBN: 1-4101-0151-7

Reprinted from the 1980 edition

Fredonia Books
Amsterdam, The Netherlands
http://www.fredoniabooks.com

Table of Contents

page

Preface

Chapter 1, Introduction   1

Chapter 2, Energy Sources   4

Chapter 3, Muscular Strength and Endurance   12

Chapter 4, Cardiovascular Fitness   42

Chapter 5, Body Composition   93

Chapter 6, Flexibility   104

Chapter 7, Exercise Precautions and Contraindications   119

Chapter 8, Getting Started   179

Tables

Table		page
1	Various Sports and Their Predominant Energy System (S)*	9
2	Arrangement of Exercises in Strength Training	21
3	Example of a Basic Isotonic Strength Training Program	30
4	Starting Weights Based on Body Weight	31
5	Example of a Basic Isometric Strength Training Program	34
6	Aerobic Capacity Classification Based on Sex and Age	44
7	Norms for 12-Minute Walking/Running Test*[a]	45
8	Norms for 1.5 Mile Run Test*	46
9	Summary of Findings from Aerobic Training Studies	48
10	Incidence of Injury with Training*	51
11	Novice Jogging Program*	52
12	Starter Jogging Program	53
13	Age-Predicted Maximum Heart Rate and Training Zone for Submaximal Exercise	57
14	Progression for Intermediate Runners	60
15	Make-up Progression for Missed Training Sessions	62
16	Energy Cost of Selected Activities	65
17	Energy Cost of Walking*	67
18	Aerobic Point Value of Selected Activities*	68
19	Energy Cost of Running*	69
20	Energy Cost of Cycling*	72
21	Physiological Changes with a Season of Intercollegiate Basketball*	79
22	Aerobic Capacity of Male Participants in Selected Athletic Events	80
23	Changes in Aerobic Capacity with De-Training: Jim Ryun, A Case Study*	86

Table		page
24	Alternative Aerobic Training Activities	83
25	Relationship Between Aerobic Capacity and Aerobic Point Performance*	89
26	Body Fat Composition	103
27	Ratings for Running Shoes*	122
28	Guidelines for Running in Cold Weather*	127
29	Guidelines for Exercise in the Heat*	134
30	A Guide for Salt Replacement*	140
31	Guidelines for the Drinking Athlete*	141
32	Abdominal Exercises	162
33	Aerobic Training Program Based on VO_2 Max	182
34	Beginning Swimming Program	184
35	Beginning Stationary Cycling Program	185
36	Beginning Cycling Program	186
37	Rope Skipping Program (80 RPM)	187
38	Normative 1-RM Data[a, b]*	190
39	Sit-up Program	192
40	Chins-YoYo Procedure	193
41	Chinning Program	194
42	Flexibility Norms*	196
43	Record Forms for Skinfold Data	200
44	Table to Convert Density to Percent Fat[a]	201
45	Assessing Body Build*	202

Illustrations

Figure   page

1   Energy Continuum   8

2   The Energy Continuum and Sports Activities*   10

3   Relationship Between Load and Speed of Contraction*   16

4   Variation in Strength Relative to Angle of Contraction with 100 Percent Representing the Angle Where Strength is Maximal   23

5   Sample Circuit Training Program   27

6   Isometric Training and Joint Angle Specificity*   33

7   Effects of Different Training Frequencies on Maximum Oxygen Uptake*   49

8   Relationship Between Heart Rate and Oxygen Uptake*   55

9   Karvonen Formula for Determination of Target Heart Rate*   58

10   Effect of Different Modes of Training on Aerobic Capacity   64

11   Energy Cost of Running vs Cycling   73

12   Age and Trainability*   91

13   Neck, Shoulder and Back Exercises   106-107

14   Causes of Low Back Pain*   109

15   Hamstring Length and Low Back Pain*   111

16   Low Back Exercises   112

17   Morning Stretching Exercises   114

18   Stretching Continuum*   117

19   Heat Safety Index*   129

20   Heat, Activity and Core Temperature   132

21   Effect of Dehydration on Heart Rate and Rectal Temperature During Two Hours of Cycling*   136

22   Effect of Glucose Concentration in a Solution on the Rate of Gastric Emptying*   138

Illustrations cont.   p. 2

Figure   page

23   Altitude and Aerobic Capacity   143

24   Exercises for the Ankle and Calf   151

25   Remedial Exercise for Shin Splints   152

26   Anatomy of Knee and Patella*   156

27   Quadricep Exercises   158

28   Stretching Exercises for Iliotibial Band Syndrome   159

29   Abdominal Exercises   161

30   Warm-up Exercises for Strength Training   168

31   Warm-up Exercises for Basketball   169-170

32   Warm-up Exercises for Cycling   171-172

33   Warm-up Exercises for Golf   173

34   Warm-up Exercises for Tennis, Racquetball and Handball   174-175

35   Warm-up Exercises for Running   176

36   Stretching Exercises for Work and/or Travel   177

37   Stretching Exercises Before Bedtime or TV   198

Appendix

		page
Appendix A	The Fast Food Calorie Counter	204-208
Appendix B	Strength Training Procedures-Free Weights	209-213
Appendix C	Strength Training Procedures-Universal Gym	214-216
Appendix D	Nautilus Training Principles	217-233

PREFACE

The purpose of this text is to use existing scientific information from
previous space flights, space medicine, exercise physiology and sports medicine to
prepare a physical fitness manual suitable for use by members of the NASA astronaut
population. With the possibility of repeated flights and numerous, diverse, in-flight
tasks, the time available for pre-flight conditioning must be utilized as effectively
as possible. For the first time, crew members will come from diverse backgrounds
and interests. The objective of this text is to provide a variety of scientifically
valid exercise programs/activities suitable for the development of physical fitness.

An attempt has been made to present programs, activities and supportive
scientific data in a concise, easy to read format so as to permit the user to select
his or her mode of training with confidence and devote time previously spent experi-
menting with training routines to preparation for space flight. The programs and
activities included in this text have been tested and shown to be effective and
enjoyable.

CHAPTER 1
INTRODUCTION

The United States is in the midst of a fitness boom. Recent articles in
prestigeous news and business journals such as Time, Newsweek, Fortune and Esquire
have exhalted the virtues of fitness and catagorized the number of fitness participants. In addition, we have witnessed a surge in the popularity of books related
to fitness, diet and health. Books such as Aerobics, New Aerobics, Aerobics for
Women and The Aerobics Way have sold several million copies and sales of magazines
such as Inside Running, The Runner and Runner's World are spiralling. James Fixx's
The Complete Book of Running has been a Book of the Month Club selection and the
nation's number 1 best selling non-fiction book.

America's infatuation with health and fitness has become big business.
Statistics indicate that U.S. citizens spend billions of dollars annually on fitness
items such as books, magazines, clothing, running shoes and athletic equipment. While
the reasons for these expenditures are numerous, research suggests that most individuals are concerned with a desire to improve personal health, avoid chronic heart
disease and/or improve physical appearance.

Individuals, however, are not alone in their desire to enhance fitness. Recently
big business has become aware of the importance of personal fitness and currently
over 300 major corporations in the U.S. spend approximately six billion dollars on
programs designed to enhance the health and fitness of their employees (Wilson, et al,
1979). Employer concern for fitness; however, is not completely altruistic.
Business has realized that a fit working/management force exhibits more stamina, fewer
acute and chronic disabling ailments, less absenteeism and more productivity (Keelor,
1979;Provasudov, 1975).

While scientific data concerning the positive effects of fitness on productivity
in the U.S. is lacking, current research does suggest that the nation's interest in

physical fitness has had positive effects on the health and fitness of its citizens. Recent data from the American Heart Association (1979) indicate that for the first time in more than a decade, America is seeing a plateau in the incidence of coronary heart disease related deaths. While the data are inconclusive to date, several researchers (Fox and Haskell, 1968; Cooper, 1978; Cooper, et al, 1976; Paffenberger and Hale, 1975; Bassler, 1975) speculate that this decline is associated with the recent increased interest in health and fitness. Hopefully, time will prove that fit individuals experience a lower incidence of coronary deaths and disabling injuries.

While American public interest in fitness has mushroomed only in the last 5-10 years, the National Aeronautics and Space Administration (NASA) has been involved with fitness since the 50's (Beischer and Fregly, 1961). NASA's initial interest in fitness was associated with a concern for the safety and welfare of crewmen. NASA flight medicine and life science personnel were concerned with preparing crewmen to meet "New Frontiers," i.e., withstand the stresses of training, lift-off, prolonged sedentary existence at zero-g, re-entry and splash-down. Using bed rest data and limited experience at zero-g, NASA personnel formulated an effective training program for early astronauts.

The success of Mercury suggested that man could indeed survive space flight and tolerate brief (Link, 1965) exposures to weightless environment. Armed with Mercury data and the results of additional bed rest studies (Miller, et al, 1965; Saltin, et al 1968), NASA personnel hypothesized that much of the physiological deterioration associated with existence at zero-g could be reduced or counteracted by in-flight exercise. Subsequent research on Apollo (Johnson, et al, 1975) and Skylab missions (Johnson and Dietlein, 1977) verified this original hypothesis. Beginning with Apollo, each mission was longer than the previous one and the amount of attention devoted to in-flight exercise was progressively increased. The results were as expected, i.e., in-flight exercise enabled man to tolerate exposures to weightlessness for periods

of time up to 84 days (Skylab 4). Skylab data (Rummel, et al, 1975; Sawin, et al,
suggested that the greater the emphasis on in-flight exercise, the less severe the
effects of flight.

Today, the emphasis has shifted. Astronauts are currently preparing for the
"Second New Frontier." We are in the era of Space Shuttle, a re-usable spacecraft
that is conducive to repeated flights of shorter duration. With the advent of
re-usable spacecraft, the possibility of repeated or multiple flights by crewmen
truly exists. Attention must be devoted to the task of developing fitness levels
sufficient to survive repeated exposures to zero-g and to ensure maintenance of fitn
levels sufficient to successfully perform physical tasks in space.

CHAPTER 2
ENERGY SOURCES

Physical Fitness; How Much Do You Need.

Traditionally, physical fitness has been defined as the ability to carry-out daily tasks (work) with vigor and alertness, without undue fatigue and with ample energy to enjoy leisure time pursuits and to meet unforeseen emergencies. Most experts have suggested that physical fitness is an individual matter. That is, the minimal level necessary will vary according to the needs of the individual.

While this definition has been advocated by authorities for at least 50 years, it is inadequate by today's standards. Using this definition, almost anyone can classify himself as being physically fit. In today's technological society, an extremely high level of fitness may not be necessary in order to earn our daily bread. However, regular physical activity is essential if the body is to function properly. Medical research suggests that an inverse relationship exists between fitness and hypokinetic disease. Hypokinetic diseases are those chronic degenerative conditions such as, stiff joints, back ache, bursitis, fatigue, poor circulation, constipation, muscle atrophy and abnormal heart conditions, that limit productivity and reduce the quality of life.

Research suggests that individuals who have a low level of fitness have a high resting heart rate, elevated blood pressure, high levels of cholesterol and tri-glyceride, are constantly fatigued, constantly out of breath and have a risk of dying from heart attack approximately 2 to 3 times greater than that of more fit colleagues. In contrast, fit individuals have less fat, a lower incidence of diabetes, gout, heart attack and lung disease, experience more restful sleep, have a lower rate of absenteeism and have more stamina for work, recreation and family activities.

In light of the aforementioned information, most authorities currently define fitness as the capacity of the heart, blood vessels, lungs and muscles to function at optimal efficiency. Optimal efficiency implies a level of muscular strength, muscular endurance, flexibility and cardiorespiratory efficiency sufficient to complete daily work, enjoy leisure pursuits, meet emergencies and prevent the development of chronic degenerative diseases. In addition to these components, body composition is an important consideration because the amount of body fat carried will affect physical performance and health status. An extensive discussion of each of these components of fitness is presented in subsequent chapters.

Energy For Muscular Work.

The energy liberated during the breakdown of foods (carbohydrates, fats and proteins) is not directly used to perform mechanical work. Rather, it is used to produce the chemical compound, adenosine triphosphate (ATP). ATP is the only source of energy available to the muscle cells to perform physical work. It is formed primarily in the mitochondria (small structures approximately the size of bacteria, which are present in the cytoplasm of cells) and stored in most cells of the body. When the cells require energy, they obtain it by splitting stored ATP molecules.

ATP Stores With The Body.

The principle storage depot for ATP is located within the individual muscle cells. Research by Hultman (1967) and Karlsson (1971) suggests that human muscle contains approximately 4-6 mM of ATP per kilogram of muscle tissue. In most individuals, this supply would be exhausted within 2 to 3 seconds of maximal effort and would have to be replaced before work could continue. The reconstruction at ATP can occur during both aerobic and anaerobic metabolism.

The quickest method of providing ATP is via anaerobic metabolism. Two methods or pathways for anaerobic metabolism of ATP exist. The first and simplest anaerobic source of ATP is called the ATP-PC pathway or system. Phosphocreatine (PC), like

ATP, is stored in the muscle cells. Muscle tissue contains approximately three times more PC (15-17 mM/kg) than ATP. When ATP is broken down during muscular contraction, it is quickly reformed from energy liberated from the breakdown of stored PC. The ATP-PC system is used to provide fuel for activities involving quick powerful bursts of activity, e.g., starting, stopping, sprinting, jumping, throwing, etc. This system is not dependent upon a series of chemical reactions nor on oxygen. Thus, it represents the most rapid source of ATP for muscle use.

The capacity of the ATP-PC system to sustain maximal effort is usually exhausted in 10 to 15 seconds. At this point, the participant has 3 choices. He can 1) stop and rest; 2) reduce the intensity to a submaximal level or 3) attempt to continue at the present pace. The first two procedures will utilize the aerobic pathway to rebuild ATP while the latter will use a second anaerobic energy source.

The second anaerobic source of ATP is called the lactic acid pathway or system. This system metabolizes the glycogen stored in the muscle cells to produce ATP. The process is called glycolysis (the dissolving of sugar) and takes place in the absence of oxygen. Without oxygen, the sugar is only partially broken down by a series of complicated chemical reactions. The end products of glycolysis are ATP (energy) and lactic acid.

The lactic acid system is a valuable source of ATP. It does, however, have serious limitations. First, lactic acid is a principle source of fatigue. Second, it is not an efficient source of ATP. Glycolysis of 1 molecule of glucose yields 2 molecules of ATP, less than 5 percent of the total yield possible via aerobic metabolism. The capacity of this system is usually exhausted in 2 to 3 minutes. Although its supply of energy is limited and brief, the lactic acid system is an extremely important source of ATP to support activities such as all-out sprints of 200-800 meters and to sustain near maximal efforts of 30 seconds to 3 minutes duration

The third source of energy is the oxygen transport (O_2) or aerobic system which is essential for sustaining submaximal efforts. In activities such as walking, jogging, swimming, cycling, etc., ATP is constantly produced via the aerobic metabolism of fats, proteins and carbohydrates. The aerobic pathway is a slow, extremely large source of ATP, providing approximately 50 times more ATP than the aforementioned anaerobic sources. Since the byproducts of the aerobic pathway are carbon dioxide and water, they are easily eliminated via breathing and perspiration and there is no build-up of waste products. This system is essential for long term (endurance) exercises performed at submaximal rates and is the principle component of cardiorespiratory or endurance fitness.

Although each system has been presented as being functionally independent, they do, in fact, overlap and individuals simultaneously utilize both anaerobic and aerobic pathways. One should think in terms of an energy continuum as depicted in Figure 1. This figure indicates that all three energy sources contribute to the production and supply of ATP during physical activity. The light and shaded areas in this figure depict the relative importance of each source. At one end of the continuum are activities of intense effort and extremely short duration. These activities are anaerobic and utilize predominantly the ATP-PC system. At the opposite end of the continuum are activities requiring submaximal effort over long periods of time. These activities utilize and develop the oxygen transport system. Near the middle is the gray zone depicting activities that utilize approximately equal amounts of aerobic and anaerobic sources. Research suggests that the gray zone exists for events lasting from 3:45 to 9:00 minutes in duration. Events to the left of the zone are predominantly anaerobic and the ones to the right are predominantly aerobic.

Mathews and Fox (1976, 1979) have constructed guidelines based upon performance time with which an individual can determine the major energy system(s) involved during the performance of any activity. Inspection of Table 1 indicates that activities requiring performance times equal to or less than 30 seconds in duration utilize and develop the ATP-PC system. Activities requiring 30 to 90 seconds for completion utilize both the ATP- PC and LA systems. Events lasting 90 to 180 seconds

FIGURE 1

ENERGY CONTINUUM*

PRIMARY ENERGY SOURCES

	ATP-PC and Lactic Acid Systems			Lactic Acid, and Oxygen Systems			ATP-PC	Oxygen System		
% Aerobic	0	10	20	30	40	50	60	70	80	90	100
% Anaerobic	100	90	80	70	60	50	40	30	20	10	0
Event (Meters)	100	200	400	800		1500	3200 (2 Miles)		5000	10,000	42,200 (Marathon)
Time (Min:Sec)	0:10	0:20	0:45	1:45		3:45	9:00		14:00	29:00	135:00

thews and Fox (1976)

TABLE 1

VARIOUS SPORTS AND THEIR
PREDOMINANT ENERGY SYSTEM (S)*

SPORTS OR SPORT ACTIVITY	% Emphasis According to Energy Systems		
	ATP-PC and LA	LA-O_2	O_2
1. Baseball	80	20	--
2. Basketball	85	15	--
3. Fencing	90	10	--
4. Field Hockey	60	20	20
5. Football	90	10	--
6. Golf	95	5	--
7. Gymnastics	90	10	--
8. Ice Hockey			
a. forwards, defense	80	20	--
b. goalie	95	5	--
9. Lacrosse			
a. goalie, defense, attack men	80	20	--
b. midfielders, man-down	60	20	20
10. Rowing	20	30	50
11. Skiing			
a. slalom, jumping, downhill	80	20	--
b. cross-country	--	5	95
c. pleasure skiing	34	33	33
12. Soccer			
a. goalie, wings, strikers	80	20	--
b. halfbacks, or link men	60	20	20
13. Swimming and diving			
a. 50 yds., diving	98	2	--
b. 100 yds.	80	15	5
c. 200 yds.	30	65	5
d. 400, 500 yds.	20	40	40
e. 1500, 1650 yds.	10	20	70
14. Tennis	70	20	10
15. Track and field			
a. 100, 220 yds.	98	2	--
b. field events	90	10	--
c. 440 yds.	80	15	5
d. 880 yds.	30	65	5
e. 1 mile	20	55	25
f. 2 miles	20	40	40
g. 3 miles	10	20	70
h. 6 miles (cross-country)	5	15	80
i. marathon	--	5	95
16. Volleyball	90	10	--
17. Wrestling	90	10	--

Mathews and Fox (1976)

FIGURE 2

THE ENERGY CONTINUUM AND SPORTS ACTIVITIES*

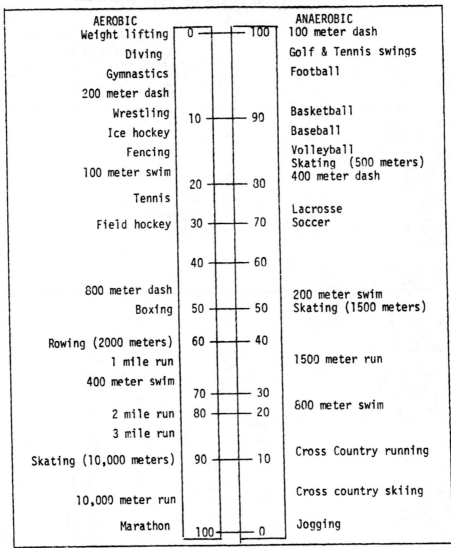

utilize the lactic acid and the oxygen transport systems and activities requiring performance times greater than 3 minutes in duration utilize the oxygen transport system. Utilizing the information in Table 1 and Figure 1, an individual can determine the predominant energy pathway used in a variety of athletic events and select a(n) activity(s) that are optimal for his/her training needs.

Physical Fitness: Sports vs Aerobic Activities.

Training is specific. The energy system used in exercise is the energy system trained or developed. Inspection of Figure 2 indicates that sports such as golf, tennis, racquetball, basketball, volleyball, etc. are predominately anaerobic in nature. These activities require skills such as starting, stopping, running, jumping and throwing - all of which are short, high intensity movements performed intermittently over the time of the game. Although these games may last 30 to 90 minutes, the specific skills required for performance are largely anaerobic. Thus, the aerobic benefits derived are minimal when compared to those resulting from activities such as, running, cycling and swimming. Cooper (1978) estimates that you would have to play over an hour of tennis singles and at least 35 continuous minutes of racquetball or basketball to achieve an aerobic training effect equivalent to that produced by running a mile in 8 minutes. Activities such as running, cycling and swimming are predominately aerobic in nature. They are more effective (large gains) and more efficient (more gains per unit of time) than team and individual sports in developing cardiorespiratory fitness.

CHAPTER 3
MUSCULAR STRENGTH AND ENDURANCE

Muscular strength is the ability of the body or its segments to apply force.
The stronger the individual, the more force that he or she can generate. Muscular
endurance is the ability to exert force repeatedly or to sustain a contraction
against moderate resistance. Chins, sit-ups and the flexed-arm hang are examples of
tests of muscular endurance. Muscular power, the ability to exert force over time,
is a function of muscular strength and speed. Power is usually thought of in
terms of explosive force and is illustrated in activities such as the vertical jump,
golf swing and tennis serve. While strength, endurance and power are often presented
as being pure components, they are functionally related during human performance and
mutually dependent upon the strength level of the participant. For example, in
events such as the shot-putt, the principle component, power, is the product of
muscular force times velocity. Increased strength will enhance the ability to
apply force and thereby contribute to power. In activities involving muscular
endurance, i.e., where an individual is required to move a fixed load through a range
of motion (chins) a given number of times, an increase in muscular strength would
enable the participant to move the load with less effort and perform more repetitions
of the activity.

Muscular Endurance vs Cardiorespiratory Endurance.

Muscular endurance refers to the ability to perform repeated muscular contractions using a specific muscle or group of muscles. Muscular endurance, also called
local endurance, is limited by the ability of the muscle or muscle groups to utilize
the anaerobic sources of energy. Energy for repeated contractions of isolated muscles
or muscle groups is derived from the existing stores of ATP-PC within the muscle and
the metabolism (glycogenesis) of glycogen. Cardiorespiratory   endurance refers to
activities involving gross or total body movement, such as running, cycling or

swimming. In gross body movements, the energy is provided by the aerobic pathway
and performance is limited by the capacity and efficiency of the respiratory,
circulatory and thermoregulatory systems.

The Overload Principle.

The overload principle states that when a system of the body is exercised at
a level above that at which it normally operates, the system will adapt and function
more efficiently. In strength training, the use of heavy resistances, i.e., resistances exceeding those normally encountered,forces the muscle to contract at maximal
or near maximal levels and thus stimulates the physiological adaptations that lead
to increases in both muscular strength and size. As a muscle increases in strength,
the initial training resistance ceases to overload the exercising muscle and thus
becomes ineffective for producing additional strength gains. Continued work with
this resistance will enable the participant to maintain a constant level of strength
but will not produce additional increases in strength. Further increases in strength
require that the muscle be overloaded throughout the course of the strength training
program. The process of periodically overloading the muscle as it adapts to the
previous workload is called progressive resistance training.

Research indicates that muscular strength can be increased through a variety
of training methods. The key to muscular development; however, is the intensity of
the work required during the exercise session. In order for training to occur, the
overload principle must be satisfied (De Lorme, 1945; De Lorme and Watkins, 1948).

The principle of progressive resistance exercise implies that strength cannot
be increased by lifting light to moderate workloads. The muscle must constantly
attempt the momentarily impossible. Attempting to lift maximal or near maximal loads
causes the body to utilize its reserve ability. The utilization of this reserve
ability is the essential factor in stimulating muscular growth.

Increasing the Workload.

In most strength training routines, the participant performs a set number of repetitions of a given exercise with a pre-determined workload. A typical example for an exercise utilizing the bench press maneuver might consist of 10 repetitions with 100 pounds of weight. This 100-pound workload is referred to as the 10-RM (10 repetition maximum). A 10-RM is a load that can be lifted correctly only ten times before fatigue sets in. During each training session, the participant should lift the 100-pound load at least 10 times. As the body adjusts to the workload, muscular strength increases and the participant is able to perform more than 10 repetitions with the 100-pound load. The participant should now strive to lift the 100-pound load as many times as possible during each workout. Whenever it is possible to lift the 100-pound load 14 times, the load should be increased by 5 to 10 pounds or until only 10 repetitions can be completed. This process should be repeated throughout training to ensure that the muscle is always adequately overloaded.

Heavy or Light Weights; Fast vs Slow Contractions.

The most important factor in strength training is the resistance imposed upon the muscle. Regardless of contractile speed, if the muscle is repeatedly contracting with a load that is easily moved, the intensity of the effort is low (submaximal) and the energy requirements are provided through aerobic metabolism. As the resistance increases, oxygen can not be provided fast enough to sustain effort and the muscles must rely on anaerobic pathways for energy. The level of work at which the body must switch from aerobic to anaerobic pathways for energy supplies is called the anaerobic threshold. Current research (Wilmore, 1976) indicates that the body must be pushed past the anaerobic threshold in order for beneficial changes to occur. Therefore, in order to improve the size, strength and function of the musculature system, work must be performed with heavy weight loads.

Inspection of the force velocity curve in Figure 3 (Lamb, 1978) indicates that velocity (speed of limb movement) decreases as the resistance to movement increases. Likewise, a decrease in resistance reduces the intensity of the work and permits a faster rate of movement. Thus, high intensity work loads, i.e., those sufficient to cause the body to reach the anaerobic threshold and stimulate growth are associated with slower rates of muscular contraction. Lighter workloads which permit rapid rates of contraction are insufficient for producing changes in muscular strength.

In addition to the aforementioned physiological reasons for using high resistance slow repetition workloads, valid biomechanical reasons exist to discourage the use of rapid muscular contractions. First, with any muscular contraction, the initial force output is used to accellerate the limb and resistance imposed. Attempts to rapidly move (accellerate) moderate tb heavy loads will produce a level of force approximately 3 to 4 times the actual workload. This force is directed to the muscles, tendons and joints of the involved limb(s) and creates a potential hazard for the musculo-skeletal system. Second, once inertia has been overcome and the resistance (barbell) begins to accellerate, the resistance (barbell) develops momentum and is in effect flying away from the working limb(s). The resulting resistance applied to the muscular system at the middle of the range of motion is negligible. Finally, at the end of the range of motion, the movement (momentum) of the barbell is checked by contraction of the antagonists which creates another potential hazard for the musculo-skeletal system. Thus, the practice of jerking a weight in an attempt to improve muscular strength through rapid contractions is dangerous and unproductive.

Regardless of the type of strength training used, training should be slow and deliberate. Participants should take 1 to 1.5 seconds to raise the resistance and approximately 2 seconds to lower it. An effective rate of movement is 100 degrees per second to raise the load and 80 degrees per second to lower it. Contractions should be smooth and deliberate. Jerky movements should be eliminated. The key to strength training is intensity. Workloads of 70 to 80 percent of maximum will ensure

FIGURE 3

RELATIONSHIP BETWEEN LOAD AND SPEED
OF CONTRACTION*

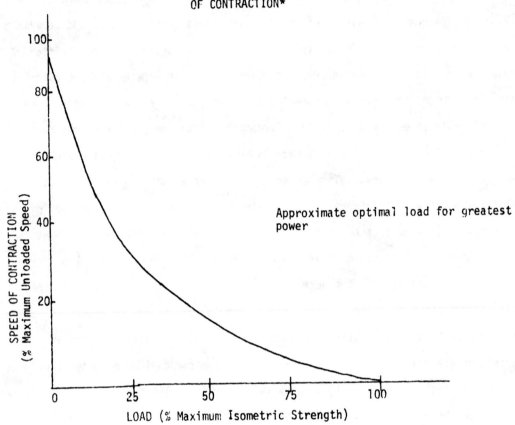

* (Lamb, 1978)

that the training intensity is above the anaerobic threshold. Ten to 15 repetitions of each exercise should be performed each training session.

Fast-twitch and Slow-twitch Muscle Fibers and Their Relationship to Strength Training.

Within the past decade, several prominent scientists (Dubowitz and Brooks, 1973) have analyzed muscle biopsies with electron microscopes and determined that at least 8 different types of muscle fibers exist within animal and mammalian skeletal muscle. Although controversy exists concerning the exact number and appropriate classification of fiber types in man, a common, but questionable practice is to classify muscle fibers as being either fast of slow-twitch. Individuals who adhere to this practice contend that fast-twitch or white fibers are biochemically suited for anaerobic activities involving speed and power. Conversely, red or slow-twitch fibers are usually associated with aerobic or endurance-type activities. Proponents of the two-fiber theory advocate separate training programs for fast-twitch and slow-twitch fibers. In general, they advocate moderate repetition, high resistance, rapid contractions for fast-twitch training and high repetition, low resistance, slow contractions for slow-twitch development.

Specific fallacies in the two-fiber theory exist. First, it is not possible to alter the ratio of fast to slow-twitch fibers with training (Gollnick, et al, 1972 and 1973; Baldwin, et al, 1972). Second, the size-principle phenomenon advocated by Costill (1979) suggests that training programs using rapid movements (rates of contraction) sitmulate slow-twitch rather than fast-twitch activity. Each muscle fiber within the human body functionally belongs to a motor unit. The motor unit, the functional unit of voluntary skeletal muscle, is composed of a motor nerve and all the muscle fibers innervated by that alpha-motoneuron. Each fiber within any one motor unit has similar physiological, biochemical and morphological properties. When a motoneuron transmits an impulse from the spinal cord to the muscle fiber it innervates, all of the muscle fibers within a specific motor unit contract. Motor units differ in regard to speed, force and endurance (i.e., length of time a muscle fiber can contract without loss of tension). Some motor units can reach a peak tension twice as fast (fast-twitch) as other units (slow-twitch). Likewise, some motor units contain larger muscle fibers capable of producing a higher level of contractile force. These high force fibers are usually fast-twitch and are innervated by the larger motoneurons. The motor units that produce the lowest force are innervated by smaller motoneurons, which have slow transmitting axons and slow contracting fibers. These slow-twitch units are usually more resistant to fatigue than most fast-twitch units.

Finally, the ratio of fast to slow-twitch fibers is not always consistent, i.e., world class athletes in power events do not all have a high ratio of fast-twitch fibers and endurance athletes do not always have a dominance of slow-twitch fibers (Thorstensson, et al, 1977; Hygaard and Nielson, 1978; Tesch, et al, 1976; Costill, et al, 1976). Muscle is a mixture of fast and slow-twitch fiber types and we apparently can not selectively recruit or train specific fiber types.

According to the force-velocity curve, an individual who trains by executing rapid movements (fast contractions) must use a low resistance. Muscle fibers that produce the lowest force are slow-twitch fibers contained in the smaller motor units. Increasing the resistance, increases the number of motor units recruited, i.e., increases the number of active slow-twitch fibers and recruits fast-twitch fibers. When the load approaches maximum, the largest motor units, the fast-twitch units, are recruited. Since the load is heavy, the rate of movement must be slow. One can not selectively recruit fast-twitch fibers by moving rapidly. Increases in muscle strength are the result of slow contractions with heavy loads (fast-twitch fibers).

Alternate Day Training.

Research indicates that individuals who lift daily experience a decrease in strength after 3 to 4 weeks of daily lifting (Hettinger, 1961; Kraus, 1949; Manzer, 1947). Apparently, muscular structure can not grow if there is insufficient recovery time. Current data (Darden, 1977) indicates that there should be approximately 48 hours between training sessions. Strength training programs performed 3 days per week on alternate days will produce significant gains in strength without risking the possibility of chronic fatigue.

Increase Load or Increase Repetitions.

After 5 to 6 exercise sessions, the muscles will have adapted to the exercise and the participant will have learned the correct movements involved in each lift. The combined effect of muscular adaptation and learning will produce an increase in strength and cause the load to be sub-threshold. At this point, the resistance should be increased by approximately 5 percent and the number of repetitions should be held constant. For instance, assume that an individual is training in the bench press by performing 8 repetitions (8-RM) with a 100-pound load. As strength increases, the participant should be able to lift the 100-pound load more than 8 times. Whenever it becomes possible to perform 10-12 repetitions with the 100-pound load, the resistance should be increased by 5 percent. The new training load now becomes 105 pounds and the participant should continue as strength increases.

Number of Sets Per Session.

The answer to this question is not clear. Historically, weight lifters have advocated programs that utilize at least 2 to 3 sets of each exercise. The load in each set was usually increased by 5 to 10 percent and the number of repetitions per set was decreased by a similar amount. A typical example of such a program would have an individual perform 3-sets with a resistance equal to the 10-RM, 8-RM and 6-RM load in sets 1, 2 and 3, respectively. Recently, new theories have been advocated in which the participant is encouraged to complete only one set of each exercise. Proponents (Darden, 1977) of these theories contend that heavy resistance training is the developmental mechanism behind strength training. When an excess amount of exercise is performed, total recovery between sets and/or workouts becomes impossible. In the absence of total recovery, the muscle can not operate at an intensity sufficient to stimulate growth.

From a practical point of view, it is time consuming to perform 2-3 sets of high intensity exercise. Since high-intensity exercise must be performed slowly (force-velocity curve), the time required to complete a set of 8 to 10 repetitions would be approximately 1 minute. The energy used to sustain this activity is provided anaerobically and is replinished within approximately 3 minutes following cessation of activity. That is, the recovery time for anaerobic metabolism is approximately 3 times the length of the work interval. Approximately 9 minutes, 3 minutes of exercise and 6 minutes of recovery, would be required to correctly perform 3 sets of one specific exercise. A workout using 3 sets of 10 different lifts could require 60 to 90 minutes. Individuals training with heavy resistive exercises should consider using only one set of each exercise. This practice is effective, requires less time, ensures that the effort is threshold and protects against chronic fatigue.

Sequences of Exercises.

For best results, workouts should begin with the largest muscle group(s) and proceed down to the smallest. The reason for this arrangement is that the smaller muscles tend to fatigue sooner than large groups and might inhibit the proper overloading of the larger muscles. Each exercise session should begin with exercises for the hips and upper legs. The next body segment to be exercised should be the chest followed by exercises for the upper arms, back, posterior aspect of legs, lower legs, ankles, shoulders, posterior aspect of upper arms, abdomen, anterior aspect of upper arms and neck. In order to ensure adequate recovery between exercises, the training program should be arranged so that no two successive exercises involve the same muscle groups. For example, the bench press and overhead (military) press should not be performed in succession since they involve similar muscle groups. A sample sequence of exercises is presented in Table 2.

TABLE 2

ARRANGEMENT OF EXERCISES IN STRENGTH TRAINING

Order	Body Side	Body Regions
1	Anterior	Upper legs and hips
2	Anterior	Chest and upper arms
3	Posterior	Back, hips and upper legs
4	Posterior	Lower legs and ankles
5	Posterior	Shoulders and upper arms
6	Anterior	Abdomen
7	Anterior	Upper arms

Larger muscle groups should be exercised first. No two exercises involving the same muscle groups should follow in succession.

Isotonic, Isometric and Isokinetic Contractions.

These terms refer to three popular forms of strength training. Isotonic training involves the actual movement or lifting of a constant resistance through the range of motion of the joint or joints involved. Weight lifting is the most popular form of isotonic training. Isometric training involves exercising against a resistance greater than the muscular force that can be applied. Since the resistance is greater than the force, the muscle does not shorten, cannot overcome the resistance and no movement occurs. Pushing against a wall is an example of an isometric contraction, i.e., a considerable amount of muscular force is generated with no noticable shortening of the involved muscles or movement of the wall. Isokinetic training is a method of exercising a muscle so that the resistance to movement is determined by the force of the muscular contraction. Training is performed on an apparatus which varies or accomodates the force applied by the participant. The resistance to movement is equivalent to the force applied to the apparatus. Resistance is controlled at a fixed speed. No matter how much force is applied the resistance will not move any faster. Users of isokinetic devices attempt to perform maximal contractions as fast as possible.

During isotonic contractions, the angle (mechanical advantage) at which the muscle pulls on the bone varies at different points in the range of motion. The data presented in Figure 4 indicates that muscular force during the biceps curl is maximal at mid-range (90 degrees) and minimal at the initial and terminal points of the movement. Since the mechanical advantage is less at these extreme points, isotonic contractions with fixed loads would be near-maximal at angles of 30 to 150 degrees and submaximal at 90 degrees. Strength is the result of both contractile force and the angle of pull. Thus, the resistance to movement during isotonic contractions is not constant throughout the range of motion.

Isokinetic devices were designed to counter-act these mechanical limitations. With isokinetic training, the resistance is changed to accommodate the strength of the muscle at each point in the range of motion. Theoretically, isokinetic training

FIGURE 4

VARIATION IN STRENGTH RELATIVE TO ANGLE OF CONTRACTION WITH 100 PERCENT REPRESENTING THE ANGLE WHERE STRENGTH IS MAXIMAL*

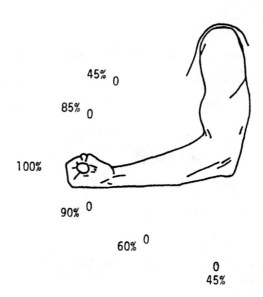

* Wilmore, 1976

permits maximal contractions of the involved muscles at each point in the range of motion. Specialized equipment such as Mini-Gym, Cybex and Nautilus are required for isotonic training. A discussion of the relative effectiveness of the various forms of strength training will be presented later.

Concentric and Eccentric Contractions.

Positive work occurs when a weight is lifted. Negative work occurs when the weight is lowered. Technical terms for positive and negative work are concentric and eccentric contractions. Concentric and eccentric refer to the type of muscular movement that occurs during exercise. Concentric contractions (positive work) occur when the muscle shortens as it develops tension. In the biceps curl, the movement of the barbell toward the chest and shoulders (upward or lifting movement) is a concentric contraction. An eccentric contraction occurs when a muscle lengthens at a controlled rate as it contracts under tension. The act of lowering a weight at a speed that acts against the force of gravity is an example of an eccentric contraction (negative work). In the biceps curl, the muscles of the upper arm increase in length as they contract eccentrically in an attempt to prevent the weight from dropping to the floor.

Recently, a considerable amount of attention has been directed toward the use of eccentric contractions. Proponents of Nautilus devices emphasize the importance of using high intensity "negative" contractions for the development of muscular strength (Darden, 1977). Since skeletal muscle can produce approximately 40 percent more tension eccentrically than concentrically , advocates of Nautilus training have theorized that greater strength gains could be produced by performing "negative" contractions with supramaximal loads. Workloads approximately 40 percent heavier than those that can be lifted concentrically are usually recommended for negative training. Scientific research; however, has failed to justify the practice of using only negative contractions. In fact, research indicates that training programs using either concentric or eccentric contractions result in nearly identical strength gains (Johnson, et al, 1976). For optimal results, one should utilize high intensity contractions emphasizing both concentric and eccentric contractions, i.e., the resistance should be lifted and lowered at a slow to moderate pace.

Muscle Soreness.

The precise cause of muscle soreness is not known. Several theories have been advanced (deVries, 1974; Hermansen, 1969; Vail, 1967). One theory suggests that lactic acid accumulates within the tissue during exercise and precipitates pain. A second theory, the spasm theory, speculates that the muscles involved in exercise go into spasms which constrict the local blood supply (ischemia) and cause pain. A third theory claims that soreness is the result of high intensity muscular forces which damage tendons and connective tissue surrounding the muscle fibers. While no universal agreement exists as to the exact cause of muscle soreness, most authorities support the latter theory. The basis for this support lies in the fact that muscle soreness is most pronounced following eccentric (negative) contractions and least pronounced following concentric (Asmussen, 1956) contractions. With high intensity negative work, the muscle lengthens under tension and stretches both the connective tissue at the muscular attachments (tendons) and the connective tissue around and within the individual muscle fibers. During concentric contractions, only the connective tissue associated with the tendons is stretched.

The degree of soreness appears to be directly related to the intensity and duration of the eccentric work performed. The onset of soreness often varies among individuals, but the severity of pain is usually greatest 24 to 48 hours after exercise. The practice of statically stretching the involved muscles before and after exercise is effective for the prevention and relief on muscle soreness. Individuals who engage in static stretching exercises while resting in a tub of hot water often find that moist heat increases circulation in the sore muscles, reduces muscle tightness, permits greater movement and significantly reduces muscle soreness.

Circuit Training.

Circuit training is the process of arranging a given number of exercises in an exercise circuit. A set number of repetitions of each exercise is performed in a given sequence. For example, a circuit may consist of the 10 exercise stations illustrated in Figure 5. The objective is to perform 10 repetitions of each exercise in sequence within an established time limit or target time. As conditioning occurs, the target time will be achieved more easily. Once this occurs, the participant must devise a method to progressively overload the working muscles. Popular methods of overloading the muscles include the use of heavier weights, increasing the number of repetitions of each exercise and/or decreasing the target time. Each variable can be manipulated separately or in combination to ensure progressive overload.

The design of the circuit (number of stations and type of exercise performed at each station) will determine which physiological parameters (strength, endurance, power, etc) are enhanced. For example, circuits consisting of weight lifting exercises produce significant increases in strength with minimal gains in cardio-respiratory endurance. Although some authorities contend that circuit training will elevate heart rate and improve cardiorespiratory fitness; this theory has not been verified by scientific study. Gettman, et al (1978) found that male police officers who performed 2 sets of a 10-station exercise circuit for 20 weeks observed significant increases in muscular strength (24 to 46 percent), but very little (3 to 5 percent) change in aerobic capacity. Similar observations were reported by Allen, et al (1976) following 12 weeks of circuit training.

Optimal Training Program for Strength Development.

Research indicates that significant increases in muscular strength will occur with isotonic, isometric and isokinetic training (Coleman, 1969; Pipes, 1978; Pipes and Wilmore, 1975; Gettman, et al, 1979). The magnitude of increase and the rate of gain appear to be independent of the mode of training as long as the training programs are similar in terms of intensity, frequency and duration (Coleman, 1969). That is,

FIGURE 5

SAMPLE CIRCUIT TRAINING PROGRAM

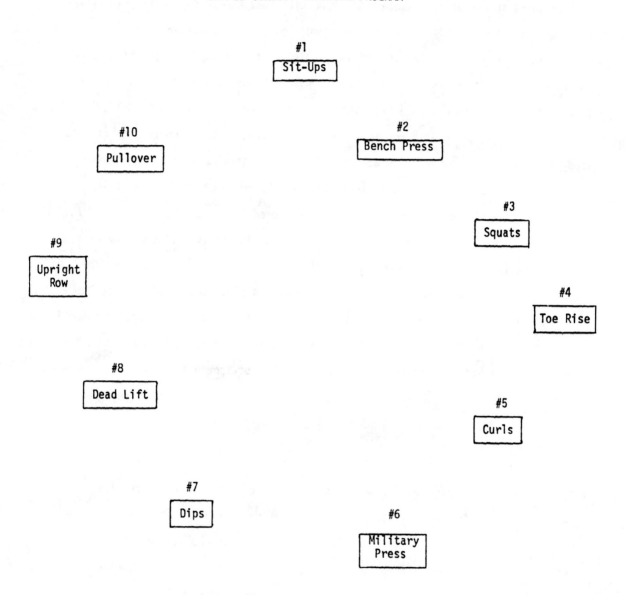

programs that utilize similar loads (RMs, sets and repetitions), at a given frequency (times per week) for a specified period of time (number of weeks) will produce similar gains in muscular strength. Discrepancies that appear in the literature are often attributable to differences in one or more of the aforementioned variables.

Recently, considerable attention has been given to a study in which high speed isokinetic training (three sets, 15 repetitions at 126 degrees per second) was found to be significantly superior to isotonic training (three sets with an 8-RM load) for the development of muscular strength (Pipes and Wilmore, 1975). The results of this study have been cited by the manufacturer of a popular isokinetic training device (Mini-Gym) flown on Skylab as being indicative of the superiority of isokinetic training. These claims; however, are being questioned. Recently, one member of the investigative team has expressed serious doubt concerning the validity of the data cited in the isokinetic study and has requested that his name be removed from the study (Wilmore, 1979). The principal investigator has proclaimed that the results have been misinterpreted and contends that the key to strength development is intensity, not speed of training. Until additional scientific data become available, it is best to assume that training programs (isotonic, isometric or isokinetic) similar in intensity, frequency and duration will produce comparable results in muscle strength.

Optimal Program for Isotonic Training.

Isotonic programs usually utilize free weights (barbells) or weight machines (Universal Gym). The optimal program consists of 1 to 3 sets of each exercise with a weight load of 2 to 10 RM, lifted three times per week on alternate days. At the beginning of the program, it is advisable to use fewer sets and lighter loads in order to allow the musculoskeletal system to gradually adapt to the stresses of training. As adaptation occurs, more sets with heavier loads can be added. For example, during the first two weeks of training, an effective program will be 1 set of exercise with a 10-12 RM load. For weeks 3 and 4, an additional set can be included (2 sets) and a 10-RM load used. After the 4th week, the participant can perform 3 sets with a load of 6 to 10 RM. The key to strength gains is the intensity of effort. Research (Berger, 1962) indicates that significant increases can occur with as little as one set of a 10-RM load. Additional gains; however, are observed with more sets (2-3 sets) and heavier loads (5-6 RM). It is important to note that it is better to perform 1 to 2 sets correctly than to rush through 3 sets. Since strength training is an anaerobic activity, sufficient recovery between sets is essential to ensure that ample energy is available for high intensity activity. As a rule of thumb, approximately 5 to 10 minutes of recovery should be permitted between sets. Sample isotonic training programs using free weights and Universal Gym are presented in Table 3.

Determining Starting Weights.

When starting a strength training program, the first requirement is the establishment of the starting loads for each exercise. The best, but most time consuming method is trial and error. For example, to determine a 10-RM load, the participant must lift several loads over a period of time in order to pin-point the load that can be lifted just 10 times to exhaustion. Since this method is time consuming, alternative methods based on body weight have been established for a few specific activities. Recommended starting weights are presented in Table 4. Additional information on the selection of starting weights is presented in Chapter 8.

Optimal Program for Isometric Training.

In isometric training the muscles contract against a fixed resistance or immovable object. Early studies (Muller and Rohmert, 1963) claimed that rapid increases in strength (approximately 5 percent per week) would occur with as few as 1 or 2, 6-second submaximal contractions. Subsequent data (Cotton, 1967; Mathews and Kraus, 1957 however, suggest otherwise. Recent investigations (Meyers, 1967; Rarick and Larsen, 1958; Rasch, 1961) indicate that increases in muscular strength are more pronounced when the participant performs several contractions against maximal resistance. In addition, evidence (Meyers, 1967) indicates that strength developed through isometric

TABLE 3 EXAMPLE OF A BASIC ISOTONIC
STRENGTH TRAINING PROGRAM

Frequency	3-4 days per week on alternate days
Duration	10-20 weeks
Sets	1-3
Load-Repetitions	6-10 RM
Recovery	5-10 minutes between sets

MODE OF EXERCISE

Free Weights	Universal Gym
1. Squats	Leg Press
2. Stiff-legged dead lift	Lateral pull
3. Bent-armed pullover	Triceps press
4. Chins	Chins
5. Shoulder shrug	Rowing
6. Bench press	Bench Press
7. Standing Curls	Curls
8. Sit-ups	Sit-ups

TABLE 4

STARTING WEIGHTS BASED ON BODY WEIGHT

	Exercise		
Free Weight	Universal Gym	Nautilus	Suggested Starting Weight
1. Squats	Leg Press	Leg Press	one-half body weight plus 10 lb
2. Stiff-legged dead lift	Lateral pull	Behind the neck	one-third body weight plus 10 pounds
3. Bent-arm pullover	Triceps press	Triceps	one-sixth body weight
4. Chins	Chins	Chins	no weight
5. Shoulder shrug	Rowing	Double shoulder	one-third body weight
6. Bench Press	Bench Press	Decline press	one-half body weight
7. Standing curls	Curls	Biceps	one-sixth body weight
8. Sit-ups	Sit-ups	Sit-ups	no weight

training is specific to the joint angle at which the exercise is performed (Figure 6). Since increases in isometric strength are maximal only at the training angle, contractions must be performed at several angles in order to effectively improve strength over the full range of motion. In most instances, this is a definite disadvantage of isometric training. Other disadvantages of isometric training are: (1) its inability to significantly affect muscular endurance and (2) subject motivation. With isometric exercise, it is easy to exert less than maximal effort. No immediate goal exists, as contrasted with lifting a weight through a given range of motion, and therefore only the most conscientious participants derive full benefits.

On the positive side, isometric training is an effective method of improving muscular strength. Other advantages of isometric training are that it is inexpensive, requires no equipment and can be performed anywhere and at any time. Since little or no equipment is needed, the same muscles can be exercised in less time than that required for weight training. A basic isometric training program is presented in Table 5

Optimal Program for Isokinetic Training.

Isokinetic training usually occurs on one or more of the following pieces of equipment: (1) Mini-Gym; (2) Nautilus and (3) Cybex. The program used will be influenced by the specific type of equipment used. The Mini-Gym is designed to provide a variable resistance equal to the muscular force being applied. This equipment possesses a speed-governor which allows the user to pre-set the speed at which he or she wishes to exercise. Ten speed setting are marked on a rotary wheel adjacent to the load mechanism. The adjustment wheel contains ten settings. A low setting reduces the tension and permits the most rapid rate of movement while a high setting increases the resistance and permits the slowest rate of movement. When the user exerts maximal effort, the machine accellerates to the pre-set speed. As the muscle continues to contract throughout the range of motion, the speed-governing action of the machine fluctuates to accommodate the varying force exerted by the muscle. In this manner, the device loads the muscle for maximal performance throughout the

FIGURE 6

ISOMETRIC TRAINING AND JOINT ANGLE SPECIFICITY*

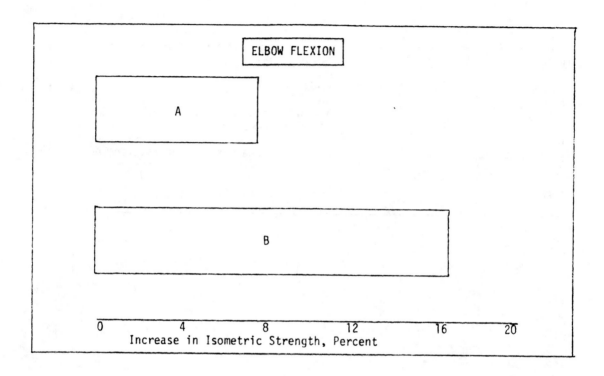

A - Training angle = 90°

B - Training angle = 170°

* Fox 1979

TABLE 5

EXAMPLE OF A BASIC

ISOMETRIC STRENGTH TRAINING PROGRAM

Frequency	4-5 days per week
Duration	10-20 weeks
Sets	3; one at each of 3 points within the normal range of motion
Load-Repetition	6-10; 6-second maximal contractions each set
Recovery	1-3 minutes between sets

range of motion once the set speed is achieved. Another advantage of this device is that it permits the user to select the speed at which he or she wishes to train. The device enables the contracting muscle to work against maximal resistance throughout the full range of motion by accommodating the varying force exerted by the muscle For example, with isotonic training involving a fixed load (RM), the load can become supra-maximal as the muscle fatigues and training must stop. With accommodating resistance, the resistance varies to accommodate the capability of the muscle at any given time or point within the range of motion. This is important in injured muscles since it will not permit the muscle to be exercised at a load above that which it can safely handle. Other advantages of the Mini-Gym include the fact that it is relatively inexpensive ($200-300), light weight (20 lbs), portable and adaptable so that several exercises can be performed on a given machine.

Disadvantages of this device are numerous. First, the 10 speed settings on the speed-governor are somewhat arbitrary. No data exist to pinpoint the exact speed of movement (RPM, or degrees/sec) for any of the 10 settings. Second, the speed of movement associated with a given speed setting will vary between different machines and within the same machine. As more repetitions are performed, the rope becomes hot and worn, thus affecting the rate of movement. Third, the principle of variable resistance allows an individual to "let-up" or exert less muscular force as he becomes fatigued or bored. An individual can exert less than maximal force on any contraction, thus producing a varying amount of muscular force. Fourth, the machine does not permit eccentric contractions. Finally, the apparatus has been observed to break when used by groups of athletes.

Individuals who use Mini-Gym devices are encouraged to use a slower setting and perform 8 to 10 maximal contractions as rapidly as possible. Maximal exertion will ensure that maximal resistance will be met throughout the complete range of motion. The principle of progressive overload can be satisfied by attempting to exert more force per contraction. A second method of ensuring progressive overload is to try to complete a set number of maximal contractions in less time, e.g., perform 10 maximal contractions in 12 seconds rather than 15. Advantages to isokinetic exercise include: (1) muscle soreness is minimal; (2) workouts require little time; (3) training is virtually injury free; (4) the apparatus is easily operated.

Nautilus equipment consists of a weight machine that employs a cam designed to compensate for the variations in force that normally occur as a muscle moves through its normal range of motion. The user of Nautilus equipment selects a resistance that he or she can handle at the starting point in the range of motion of a given exercise. As movement occurs, the machine weight remains constant, but the cam alters the movement arm of the machine and increases or decreases the resistance to match the available muscular force. The cams were designed in accordance with strength curves established for a number of muscular movements. This design ensures that the relative resistance will be lower at the weaker positions and higher at the stronger positions in each movement. Another advantage of this device is that once the weight is set, the participant must exert the same degree of effort in each contraction in order to produce movement, i.e., he can not "cheat" as he can in devices that use fixed speed and variable resistance (Mini-Gym and Cybex).

Nautilus machines are designed to place the working muscles in a stretched position at the starting point for each exercise. When the muscle is pre-stretched, a nuerological signal is sent to the brain that results in a higher percentage of the muscle being contracted. Thus, a muscle placed in a pre-stretched position will contract with greater force.

Nautilus machines permit the muscle to work both concentrically and eccentrically. In addition, specific machines have been designed to permit total negative training by allowing the user to lift a supra-maximal load with the stronger muscles of the hips and legs and then to eccentrically lower the load with the muscles of the arms and shoulders. A variety of Nautilus machines are available for strength training. In general, each machine is designed for 1 or 2 specific muscle groups and/or movement patterns.

Although Nautilus machines have been shown to be effective and are extremely popular in professional sports, college athletics and private health clubs, they are not totally void of problems. Nautilus machines are very expensive. Prices range from $800.00 to $5000.00 per machine. Since each machine is designed for 1 or 2 movements, several machines are needed for total body training. The cost of establishing several Nautilus stations is prohibitative for the average individual. Thus, individuals who utilize Nautilus machines often belong to special health/spa-type facilities or have access to special training facilities.

The Cybex is a very expensive ($8000.00-$15,000.00) isokinetic device developed for research and rehabilitation purposes. Its function is similar to that of the Mini-Gym apparatus, i.e., fixed speed and variable resistance. Although highly accurate and reliable, the instrument is not designed for multiple person use. Likewise, it's cost, design and maintenance prohibit its use for group training. The Cybex is a research instrument and is not suited for training.

Each of the aforementioned pieces of apparatus will effectively improve muscular strength. Definite advantages and limitations exist for each device. Selection of a particular device will depend upon availability and personal preference of the user. Specific weight training exercises are presented in the Appendix.

Specific Changes Occurring Within the Muscle with Training.

With training, one can expect increases in the strength, endurance and size of the working muscles. An increase in muscular size is called hypertrophy. For nearly 100 years, scientists have thought that hypertrophy was due entirely to an increase in the diameter of already existing muscle fibers. Early study failed to show any increase in fiber number with training. Recent studies with animals and humans; however, have reversed these earlier findings. Studies (Costill, 1979) involving maximal workloads indicate that the muscles of power lifters increase in both size (diameter) and number. Increases in fiber number are thought to be the result of longitudinal splitting of muscle fibers (Edington and Edgeron, 1976). Muscle hypertrophy and muscular fiber splitting are the principle, but not the sole determinants of muscle size. Other factors such as increases in myofibril number, muscle protein levels and hypertrophy of connective, tendinous and ligamentous tissue are also observed with training and contribute to post-training muscle girth (Booth and Tipton, 1970).

In addition to increases in size, trained muscles also experience metabolic alterations that influence the capacity and efficiency of the working muscles. Specific metabolic changes include increases in muscle stores of ATP (18%), PC (22%) and glycogen (66%) (Mathews and Fox, 1976).

The strength of a muscle is roughly proportional to its circumference. Research (Hettinger, 1961) indicates that a muscle can exert approximately 4 kg of force per square cm of muscle cross-sectional area. Thus, increases in muscle girth (cross-sectional area) following training should result in an increase in muscular strength. While the relationship between muscle girth and strength does exist, girth is not the sole determinant of muscular strength. Often we see individuals with impressive looking muscles who are not as strong as individuals with smaller muscles. How is this possible? First, the potential for muscular strength is determined by factors other than muscle girth. Darden (1977) contends that the primary determinant of muscular strength is the effective length of the contracting muscle, i.e., the distance between the tendonous attachments at the origin and insertion of the muscle. According to Darden (1977), an untrained muscle that is 50 percent longer than a similar untrained muscle has the potential to have 2.25 times as much cross-sectional area (1.5 X 1.5 = 2.25) and 3.375 times as much volume or mass (1.5 X 1.5 X 1.5 = 3.375). Thus, the ultimate size and strength of a given muscle is determined by the length of the muscle. Unfortunately, the length of a muscle is a function of heredity and we are unable to alter our genetic make-up.

Cessation of Training.

If training is terminated, strength is lost at a rate approximately equal to that at which it was gained (Hettinger, 1961). Strength gained rapidly over a few weeks is lost rapidly and strength gained gradually lasts longer after training. Although much of the increased strength is lost in the absence of training, a portion is retained for a long period and a small amount is retained indefinitly.

Early studies (Hettinger, 1961) suggested that, following prolonged training, the rate of strength loss could be retained with one training session every six weeks and that all the strength gained could be retained with only one training session every two weeks. More recent investigations have failed to substantiate these observations (Syster and Stull, 1970; Waldman and Stull, 1969). Research by Berger (1962) suggests that strength gained through training can be maintained with maximal contractions performed only once each week. Similar observations were reported by Guess (1967) and Coleman (1969, 1970) when subjects performed submaximal repetitions (75 to 80 percent of maximum) twice per week. Darden (1977) contends that high levels of muscular strength will begin to decrease after approximately 96 hours of inactivity and recommends that training be performed at least every fourth day. No data exist to substantiate his claims.

Often individuals will train for a period of time and then use athletics or sports as a means of maintaining muscular strength. Research data indicate that this approach is not tenable. Studies by Guess (1967), Coleman (1978) and Campbell (1967) indicate that high school, college and professional athletes experienced significant reductions in muscular strength while participating on competitive baseball and football teams. Athletes required to lift weights two days per week, in addition to sports participation, experienced no significant losses of muscular strength.

The most difficult phase in strength training occurs during the early weeks when the participant is trying to increase muscular strength and endurance. Once a sufficient level of training has been attained, it is relatively easy to maintain the newly developed gains. A sufficient level of training can be maintained by exercising with maximal loads once per week or by exercising with sub-maximal loads (75 to 80 percent) twice per week. Participation in athletics and/or team sports is ineffective for maintaining muscular strength.

Women and Strength Training.

Data exist to indicate that the typical male is considerably stronger than the average female (Drinkwater, 1973). Several studies have presented evidence to indicate that men are 30 to 40 percent stronger than women. The magnitude of difference between males and females will vary for various muscle groups (Wilmore, 1974). In terms of arm and upper body strength, women usually possess only 30 to 50 percent as much strength as males. Tests of leg strength; however, often reduce this difference to 15 to 20 percent. When strength is expressed relative to body size (weight), the strength scores for women are more similar to those of men, and when expressed relative to lean body weight, females are often as strong as men. Thus, per cross-sectional area of muscle tissue, women are as strong as men (3 to 4 kg/cm^2). No significant difference exists between the quality of muscle tissue in males and females. Observable differences are attributable to differences in body size and quanity of muscle mass. At full maturity, the average female is approximately 5 to 6 inches shorter, 30 to 40 pounds lighter, possesses 40 to 50 pounds less lean body weight and is 10-15 percent fatter than the average male.

Several studies have confirmed that women can observe significant increases in muscular strength with training. Recent research by Wilmore (1974) and Coleman (1977) has demonstrated that non-athletic young women can achieve strength gains, as large as 30 to 100 percent, following 10 to 12 weeks of training. These increases in total body strength were not accompanied by gains in muscle bulk. Thus, females can increase muscular strength without developing excessively large, bulky muscles. Composite results from several studies indicate that females observe significant losses of absolute and relative body fat, significant increases in lean body weight (muscle mass) and minimal increases in muscle girth (less than .25 inches) following weight training programs. The inability of females to experience muscle hypertrophy is due mainly to their relatively low levels of testosterone compared to males.

Changes in Body Composition Following Strength Training.

Research indicates that individuals can expect significant changes in muscle girth and body composition following strength training. Studies by Wilmore (1974) indicate that individuals participating in weight training activities will experience little or no change in total body weight, but will notice significant reductions in fat weight and significant increases in lean body mass. Lean body mass, determined by subtracting the weight of body fat from the total body weight, is sometimes called fat-free weight. This fat-free weight reflects mainly the skeletal muscle mass but also includes the weight of other tissues and organs such as bone and skin. Within the human body, approximately 40 to 50 percent of the fat-free weight is muscle mass. As body fat increases, lean weight decreases. The average lean weight of adult males is approximately 85 percent of total body weight, while that for females is approximately 75 percent of total body weight. Wilmore (1974) indicates that adult men experience significant reductions in body fat and significant increases in lean body mass following weight lifting. Similar responses should be observed following Nautilus training, circuit weight training or isokinetic training. Changes in body composition of women following strength training will parallel those reported for men.

CHAPTER 4

CARDIOVASCULAR FITNESS

Cardiorespiratory endurance, formerly called stamina, is the ability of the cardiovascular and respiratory systems to take in, transport and deliver oxygen to the tissue cells where it is combined with food stuffs to produce energy. Individuals who are capable of delivering large amounts of oxygen to the tissues are said to have a high level of aerobic capacity or endurance fitness. Aerobic fitness, unlike muscular endurance, the ability of a single muscle or group of muscles to sustain prolonged exercise, is related to the development of the cardiovascular and respiratory systems and refers to the ability of the total body to sustain prolonged, rhythmic exercise. Most authorities (Cooper, 1968; Pollock, et al, 1978) contend that cardiorespiratory endurance is the most important physical attribute that an individual can possess. Recent publications (Cooper, 1978) suggest that the terms "cardiovascular endurance" and "aerobic capacity" have become synonymous with the term "physical fitness

Assessing Cardiorespiratory Fitness.

Cardiorespiratory fitness is usually determined in a laboratory setting by having the subject pedal a bicycle ergometer or walk-run on a motor-driven treadmill to exhaustion or volitional fatigue. During the test, a physician and technicians are present to ensure the safety of the subject and to monitor special equipment designed to evaluate heart rate, ECG activity and blood pressure responses. In addition, breathing apparatus are used to collect the air expired by the participant during the work task. The air collected during the last 30 to 60 seconds of work is analyzed for volume, temperature and gas concentration (oxygen and carbon dioxide). These data are then used to calculate the metabolic work performed during the last minute of effort (Consolazio, et al, 1963). Since calculations are based on data collected during the last 30-60 seconds of exhaustive work, they reflect maximal effort and are indicative of the maximal level of metabolic work that the subject is capable of attaining. Maximal metabolic work, expressed as volume of oxygen utilized (ml/min), is technically called maximal oxygen uptake or VO_2 max. Since absolute VO_2 max (ml/minute) is related to body weight, minute volumes are usually corrected for weight and criterion values expressed in terms of mililiters of oxygen used per kilogram of body weight per minute, i.e., ml O_2/Kg/min. The higher the VO_2 max, the greater the capacity for prolonged aerobic work.

Since procedures for determining aerobic capacity in the laboratory are complex time-consuming and impractical for determining cardiorespiratory fitness in large numbers of "healthy" people, field tests have been established that correlate reasonably well with laboratory determined values for VO_2 max. Most field tests utilize walking, running or jogging. Examples of these are presented in Chapter 8.

Criterion levels of fitness based on laboratory (ml O_2/Kg/min) and field tests (time) developed by Balke (1963) and modified by Copper (1968) have been revised by other authorities (Katch and McArdle, 1977). Fitness classifications based on these findings are presented in Tables 6, 7 and 8. The data in these Tables indicate that males aged 30 to 39 years who are in good aerobic condition should have a VO_2 max of 43 to 50 ml/Kg/min and should be able to run 1.5 miles in 11:01 to 12:30.

The discrepancy between VO_2 max standards for males and females is attributable to physiological differences between the sexes. Research (Astrand, 1960; Drinkwater 1973) indicates that females have a smaller stroke volume (volume of blood ejected from the heart per beat) than males for equivalent levels of submaximal work. In addition, females have a lower concentration (-10%) of hemoglobin than males. The combined effect of reduced stroke volume and hemoglobin concentration limits the maximal cardiac output (volume of blood ejected per minute) and oxygen forwarding capacity of females. Since the heart and circulatory system transport and deliver a smaller quantity of oxygen to the tissues, the VO_2 max and endurance capacity of females are considerably less than that of males.

TABLE 6

AEROBIC CAPACITY CLASSIFICATION BASED ON SEX AND AGE

	Maximal oxygen consumption (ml/kg/min)				
Age	Low	Fair	Average	Good	High
Women					
20-29	28	29-34	35-40	41-46	47
30-39	27	38-33	34-38	39-45	46
40-49	25	26-31	30-37	38-43	44
50-65	21	22-28	27-34	35-40	41
Men					
20-29	37	38-41	42-50	51-55	56
30-39	33	34-37	38-42	43-50	51
40-49	29	30-35	36-40	41-46	47
50-59	25	26-30	31-38	39-42	43
60-69	21	22-25	26-33	34-37	38

TABLE 7

NORMS FOR 12-MINUTE WALKING/RUNNING TEST*[a]

FITNESS CATEGORY		13-19	20-29	30-39	40-49	50-59	60+
Very Poor	(men)	1.30	1.22	1.18	1.14	1.03	.87
	(women)	1.0	.96	.94	.88	.84	.78
Poor	(men)	1.30-1.37	1.22-1.31	1.18-1.30	1.14-1.24	1.03-1.16	.87-1.02
	(women)	1.00-1.18	.96-1.11	.95-1.05	.88-.98	.84-.93	.78-.86
Fair	(men)	1.38-1.56	1.32-1.49	1.31-1.45	1.25-1.39	1.17-1.30	1.03-1.20
	(women)	1.19-1.29	1.12-1.22	1.06-1.18	.99-1.11	.94-1.05	.87-.98
Good	(men)	1.57-1.72	1.50-1.64	1.46-1.56	1.40-1.53	1.31-1.44	1.21-1.32
	(women)	1.30-1.43	1.23-1.34	1.19-1.29	1.12-1.24	1.06-1.18	.99-1.09
Excellent	(men)	1.73-1.86	1.65-1.76	1.57-1.69	1.54-1.65	1.45-1.58	1.33-1.55
	(women)	1.44-1.51	1.35-1.45	1.30-1.39	1.25-1.34	1.19-1.30	1.10-1.18
Superior	(men)	1.87	1.77	1.70	1.66	1.59	1.56
	(women)	1.52	1.46	1.40	1.35	1.31	1.19

* Cooper (1977)

[a] Miles

TABLE 8

NORMS FOR 1.5 MILE RUN TEST*

Fitness Category		13-19	20-29	30-39	40-49	50-59	60+	Age
Very Poor	(men)	15:31	16:01	16:31	17:31	19:01	20:01	
	(women)	18:31	19:01	19:31	20:01	20:31	21:01	
Poor	(men)	12:11-15:30	14:01-16:00	14:44-16:30	15:36-17:30	17:01-19:00	19:01-20:00	
	(women)	18:30-16:55	19:00-18:31	19:30-19:01	20:00-19:31	20:30-20:01	21:00-21:31	
Fair	(men)	10:49-12:10	12:01-14:00	12:31-14:45	13:01-15:35	14:31-17:00	16:16-19:00	
	(women)	16:45-14:31	18:30-15:55	19:00-16:31	19:30-17:31	20:00-19:01	20:30-19:31	
Good	(men)	9:41-10:48	10:46-12:00	11:01-12:30	11:31-13:00	12:31-14:30	14:00-16:15	
	(women)	14:30-12:30	15:54-13:31	16:30-14:31	17:30-15:56	19:00-16:31	19:30-17:31	
Excellent	(men)	8:37- 9:40	9:45-10:45	10:00-11:00	10:30-11:30	11:00-12:30	11:15-13:59	
	(women)	12:29-11:50	13:30-12:30	14:30-13:00	15:55-13:45	16:30-14:30	17:30-16:30	
Superior	(men)	8:37	9:45	10:00	10:30	11:00	11:15	
	(women)	11:50	12:30	13:00	13:45	14:30	16:30	

* Cooper (1977)

Training the Cardiorespiratory System.

Recent studies indicate that most adults can improve cardiorespiratory fitness as much as 10-20 percent with training (Pollock, 1973). The magnitude of improvement is dependent upon factors such as intensity, frequency and duration of the exercise program. In addition, other factors such as initial status of health and fitness, mode of exercise (walking, running, cycling, etc), regularity of exercise and age will also influence training effectiveness. Table 9 contains a summary of pertinent findings from recent training studies related to minimal requirements necessary for optimal training of the cardiorespiratory system. These recommendations are designed for the needs of the general population, not for highly trained endurance athletes or individuals of low or poor health status.

Frequency-Duration of Effort.

Research indicates that exercise should be performed on a regular basis from 3 to 5 days per week. Training sessions performed fewer than 3 times per week generally fail to improve aerobic fitness (Pollock, 1973; Pollock, 1978; Gettman, et al, 1976). Improvement observed in beginners training 5 times per week is greater than that observed training 3 times per week, but is accompanied by a higher incidence of exercise-induced musculoskeletal injury (Pollock, et al, 1977).

Pollock, et al (1977) examined the effects of training 1, 3 or 5 days per week among males age 20-35 years who trained at 85-90 percent of maximal heart rate for 30 munutes per session for a period of 20 weeks. The results, depicted in Figure 7, indicated that oxygen uptake improved approximately 5 percent in subjects who trained only once per week. Subjects who trained 3 times per week improved approximately 13 percent while those who trained 5 times per week improved 17 percent. Similar observations have been reported by other investigators (Gettman, et al, 1976).

While the aforementioned data indicate that magnitude of gain is related to frequency of training, it is important to caution beginners against attempting too much too soon. Individuals of low aerobic fitness did not achieve this status over-

TABLE 9

SUMMARY OF FINDINGS FROM AEROBIC TRAINING STUDIES

Frequency of exercise	3 to 5 days per week
Intensity of exercise	60 to 90 percent of maximum heart rate 50 to 80 percent of maximum oxygen uptake
Duration of exercise	15 to 60 minutes, continuous
Mode of exercise	Run, walk, cycle, swim
Initial level of fitness	High - higher work load Low - lower work level

FIGURE 7
EFFECTS OF DIFFERENT TRAINING FREQUENCIES
ON MAXIMUM OXYGEN UPTAKE*

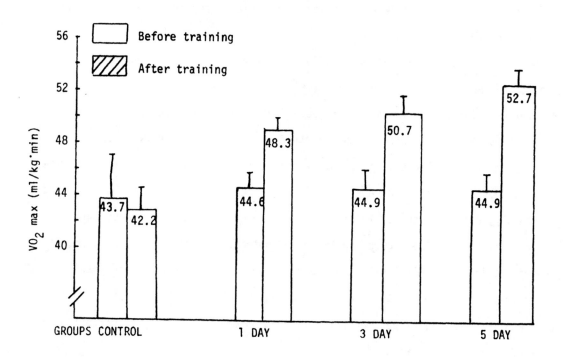

* Pollock, et al (1978)

night and will not significantly alter their status with 3 to 4 training sessions. The prudent procedure is to start slowly and gradually increase effort as your fitness level improves. Individuals who train too hard, too often and/or do not allow adequate time for recovery between training sessions are frequently injured and must cease exercise (Daniels, et al, 1977).

Pollock, et al, (1977) trained 157, 20 to 35 year old males incarcerated in state and county correctional facilities for a period of 20 weeks. Participants trained 3 days per week for 15, 30 and 45 minute durations at the state facility and for 30 minutes 1, 3 or 5 days per week at the county facility. All subjects trained at 85-90 percent of maximal heart rate. As expected, results indicated that cardiorespiratory fitness improved in direct proportion to frequency and duration of training. Unfortunately, attrition due to injury was also directly related to frequency and duration of training. The figures in Table 10 indicate that the injury rate among beginners who jogged 45-minutes per day, 3 times per week was approximately twice that of colleagues who trained 15 to 30 minutes per day. Likewise, 40 percent of novice joggers who trained 5 times per week were injured as opposed to only 12 percent of those who ran 3 times per week.

The threshold level of training and injury appears to be 30 minutes per day, 3 times per week. Individuals who train longer or more frequently seek additional gains at the risk of injury. Beginners should start with short runs (15-30 minutes) on alternate days (3-4 times/week). As the musculo-skeletal system becomes conditioned the participant can gradually increase the duration and/or frequency of training runs. Recommended novice jogging programs are presented in Tables 11 and 12. The program presented in Table 11 is used by Cooper with individuals of low fitness and requires the participant to walk for 4 weeks prior to jogging. The program in Table 12 has been used with college students and university faculty and has been observed to be effective for beginners as well as intermediate and advanced runners. This program ensures early success and gradually increases the total work load as the individual's tolerance to work increases.

TABLE 10

INCIDENCE OF INJURY WITH TRAINING*

Duration of Training	
Minutes per day	Percent Injured
15	22
30	24
45	54

3 times/week for 20 weeks

Frequency of Training	
Days per week	Percent Injured
1	0
3	12
5	39

30 minutes/day for 20 weeks

* Pollock, et al (1977)

TABLE 11

NOVICE JOGGING PROGRAM*

Week	Activity	Distance (miles)	Time (min)	Frequency (days/week)
1	Walk	1.0	17-20	5
2	Walk	1.5	25-29	5
3.	Walk	2.0	32-35	5
4	Walk	2.0	28-32	5
5	Walk-Jog-Walk	2.0	27	5
6	Walk-Jog-Walk	2.0	26	5
7	Walk-Jog-Walk	2.0	25	5
8	Walk-Jog-Walk	2.0	24	5
9	Jog	2.0	23	5
10	Jog	2.0	22	5
11	Jog	2.0	21	5
12	Jog	2.0	20	5

After week 12, jog 2 miles in 20 minutes, 4 times/week

* Cooper (1980)

TABLE 12
STARTER JOGGING PROGRAM

Week	Training Jog (min)	Walk (min)	Jog (min)	Repeat (times)	Total Time (min)	Frequency
1	:30	:30	:30	6	12	4
2	1:00	:30	1:00	10	15	4
3	2:00	:30	2:00	7	18	4
4	3:00	:30	3:00	6	21	4
5	4:00	:30	4:00	5	24	4
6	5:00	:30	5:00	5	27	4
7	6:00	:30	6:00	5	30	4
8	7:00	:30	7:00	4	30	4
9	8:00	:30	8:00	4	30	4
10	9:00	:30	9:00	3	30	4
11	10:00	:30	10:00	3	30	4
12	11:00	:30	10:00	1	22	4
13	12:00	:30	8:00	1	20	4
14	13:00	:30	7:00	1	20	4
15	14:00	:30	6:00	1	20	4
16	15:00	:30	5:00	1	20	4
17	16:00	:30	4:00	1	20	4
18	17:00	:30	3:00	1	20	4
19	18:00	:30	2:00	1	20	4
20	19:00	:30	1:00	1	20	4
21	20:00	:30	——	—	20	4

<u>Intensity of Training.</u>

The most important factor in writing an exercise prescription for the improvement of cardiorespiratory fitness is the intensity of the exercise bout, i.e., how hard you have to work. While athletes are accustomed to working at maximal levels, the typical adult is neither physiologically nor psychologically prepared to tolerate such exhaustive workouts. Fortunately, recent research indicates that submaximal effort can produce significant changes in endurance capacity. The minimal threshold for training the cardiopulmonary system appears to be approximately 50-80 percent of aerobic capacity (1975). Since oxygen uptake and heart rate are linearly related at submaximal levels of work, heart rate can be used to estimate work intensity (Figure 8). A training intensity between 60 and 90 percent of age adjusted maximal heart rate appears to be optimal for improving endurance capacity.

Most authorities (Pollock, et al, 1978; Cooper, 1970) recommend heart rate as the index of stress because:

(1) It represents a simple physiological parameter that can be easily monitored by an individual and which provides meaningful insight into the degree of metabolic and myocardial stress.

(2) The linear relationship between heart rate and oxygen consumption at submaximal levels of work permits one to estimate the metabolic cost of exercise.

(3) A high correlation (r=.89) exists between heart rate, myocardial blood flow and myocardial oxygen consumption.

(4) Heart rate, in its relationship to the work of the heart, is independent of environmental factors. Thus, an individual confronted with hot, humid weather or changes in altitude, must decrease metabolic work in order to maintain a threshold heart rate.

(5) Heart rate response to a standard submaximal exercise load decreases with training, requiring progressive increases in effort to sustain a threshold rate.

Training intensity is quantified by having an individual exercise at his own, individualized training heart rate (THR). The THR is established from the results

FIGURE 8

RELATIONSHIP BETWEEN HEART RATE AND OXYGEN UPTAKE*

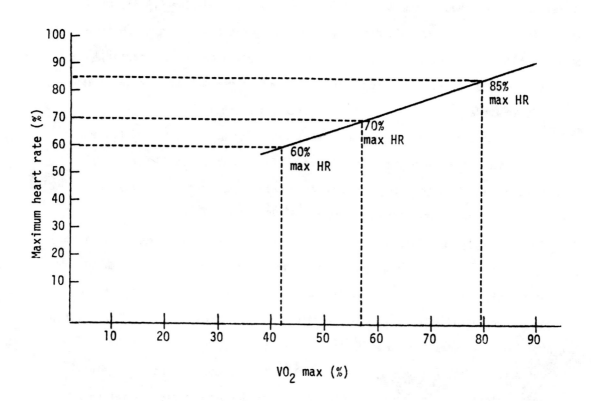

* Pollock. et al. 1978

of a maximal exercise stress test or estimated from a table of age-adjusted maximal heart rates determined for a representative population (Table 13). According to guidelines established by the American College of Sport Medicine (1975), the minimal threshold for improving aerobic capacity is a heart rate equivalent to 60 percent of maximum heart rate. Likewise, the upper-limit for safe exercise in "normal," "healthy" individuals is a rate equal to 90 percent of maximal heart rate. Heart rates within these limits are, in general, safe and effective.

The intensity that can be tolerated will vary with age, health and fitness. Marathon runners often tolerate 2 to 3 hours of running at 80 to 90 percent of maximum capacity, while most beginners cannot perform continuous effort at this level for more than a few minutes (Daniels, et al, 1978). The proper intensity level for most beginners will usually range from 60 to 70 percent of maximum for walking and between 70 and 80 percent for jogging. Intensity levels ranging from 50 to 60 percent are classified as low to moderate work. An intensity level of 70 to 80 percent is considered as moderate work and levels in excess of 90 percent of maximum are high-intensity work (American College of Sports Medicine, 1975).

While early data (Karvonen, et al, 1957) indicated that appreciable gains in cardiorespiratory fitness occur when the heart rate during exercise is raised by approximately 60 percent of the difference between resting and maximal heart rate, recent studies (Pollock, 1973) suggest that 75 percent represents a safe and more effective intensity for most "normal," "healthy" individuals. The training heart rate (THR) is calculated as follows:

(1) Maximal heart rate - resting heart rate

(2) Multiply this difference by .75

(3) Add this product to the resting heart rate

The Karvonen (1957) procedure is illustrated in Figure 9 for an individual with a maximum heart rate of 200 beats per minute.

While it is difficult to establish a single ideal intensity, previous experience suggests that an exercise level of 75 percent of HR max is best for producing significant

TABLE 13

AGE-PREDICTED MAXIMUM HEART RATE AND
TRAINING ZONE FOR SUBMAXIMAL EXERCISE

Age, Years	Age-predicted maximum heart rate	Training Sensitive Zone	
		Lower limit: 70% heart rate	Upper limit: 90% heart rate
15	210	147	189
20	200	140	180
25	195	136	175
30	190	133	171
35	185	129	166
40	180	126	162
45	173	121	156
50	166	116	149
55	160	112	144
60	155	108	139
65	150	105	135

FIGURE 9

KARVONEN FORMULA FOR DETERMINATION OF TARGET HEART RATE*

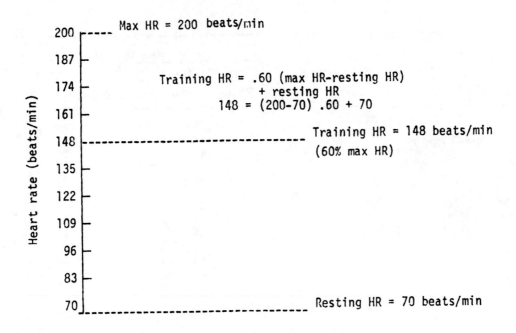

* Pollock, et al. 1978.

cardiopulmonary benefits. For most young adults, this intensity represents a THR of 150 to 170 bpm. Since maximal heart rate declines with age, a rate of 130 to 140 bpm may be sufficient for most older adults.

Novice Programs and Progressions.

The beginning program advocated by Cooper and presented in Table 11 recommends that the participant walk and/or run a given distance within a prescribed period of time. Participants are permitted to establish their own rest-work cycles. The program in Table 12 asks the participant to assess his fitness level, select the appropriate starting point and progress according to specifications depicted in the Table.

A novice, for example, would alternately jog and walk for 30 seconds. The procedure would be repeated 6 times so that the total activity period is 12 minutes in duration. This approach enables the novice to run-walk approximately one mile on the first day of training, prevents the development of signs of distress, e.g., labored breathing, stitch in the side and acidosis, and minimize the chances of musculoskeletal problems associated with over-use. After the first week, the participant increases his jog by 30 seconds while holding the walk time constant. During subsequent weeks, progress is made by increasing jog time. After approximately 15 to 16 weeks, the typical participant can run continuously for 16 minutes (approximately 1.5-2.0 miles). Further progress is made through the use of the interval training procedure depicted in Table 14.

An individual who wants to increase the duration of effort beyond 16 minutes is encouraged to run 16 minutes, walk 30 to 60 seconds and then run-walk for four, 2-minute bouts (Table 12). During the first week, he would:

```
 (1)   run 16 minutes
 (2)   walk 30-60 seconds
 (3)   run 2 minutes
 (4)   walk 30-60 seconds
 (5)   run 2 minutes
 (6)   walk 30-60 seconds
 (7)   run 2 minutes
 (8)   walk 30-60 seconds
 (9)   run 2 minutes
(10)   walk 30-60 seconds
```

TABLE 14

PROGRESSION FOR INTERMEDIATE RUNNERS

Week	Run (min)	Walk (min)	Run (min)	Walk (min)	Run (min)	Walk (min)	Run (min)	Walk (min)	Run (min)	Walk (min)	T Time (min)
1	16	1	2	1	2	1	2	1	2	1	29
2	18	1	2	1	2	1	2	1	2	1	31
3	20	1	2	1	2	1	2	1	2	1	33
4	22	1	2	1	2	1	2	1	2	1	35
5	24	1	2	1	2	1	2	1	2	1	37
6	26	1	2	1	2	1	2	1	2	1	40
7	28	1	2	1	2	1	2	1	2		40
8	30	1	2	1	2	1	2	1	1		40
9	32	1	2	1	2	1	1				40
10	34	1	2	1	2						
11	36	1	2	1							40
12	38	1	2								40
13	40										40

Using this approach, he would run within his tolerance level (16 minutes; approximately 2 miles) and then use a jog-walk pattern to progressively overload the cardio-respiratory and musculoskeletal systems. During the second week, he would run 18 minutes and then run-walk 3 additional 2-minute periods. By week 5, he would be running continuously for 24 minutes. This procedure minimizes discomfort and injury by allowing the individual to gradually increase his time and mileage as his tolerance to exercise increases.

Some individuals increase mileage by running a given distance and intervaling (jog-walk) one additional mile after each training session. An individual who wants to increase his mileage from 3 to 5 miles, for example, would run 3 miles continuously walk for 30-60 seconds and jog four, .25 mile intervals with 30-60 seconds of rest between each. During the second week, he would run 2.25 miles continuously, rest 30-60 seconds and then run-walk 4, .25 mile bouts. Using this approach, he would add .25 miles to his continuous jog each week and interval a mile after each workout. This procedure would be followed until the goal (40 minutes or approximately 5 miles in this example) is achieved (Table 14).

A modified version of this approach can be used by individuals who, because of travel and/or illness, are forced to miss 1-2 weeks of training. For example, an individual accustomed to running 2 miles per day who does not train for 7-10 days can regain his status by using the program presented in Table 15. Individuals who miss training sessions will find that this approach permits them to gradually regain their status without undue physiological or musculoskeletal stress.

Mode of Training.

Numerous studies have been conducted to determine the optimal training activity. The results indicate that training is specific, i.e., the energy system trained is the energy system developed. Aerobic activities such as jogging, swimming, etc. will do little to enhance muscular strength. Likewise, anaerobic activities such as calisthenics and weight training will be minimally effective in altering endurance fitness.

TABLE 15
MAKE-UP PROGRESSION FOR
MISSED TRAINING SESSIONS

Day	Run (miles)	Walk (sec)	Run (miles)	Walk (sec)	Repeat (times)	Total Distance (miles)
1	1.00	30-60	.25	30-60	4	2
2	1.25	30-60	.25	30-60	3	2
3	1.50	30-60	.25	30-60	2	2
4	1.75	30-60	.25	30-60	1	2
5	2.00	30-60	0	0	0	2

Attempts to compare the effectiveness of walking, running and cycling indicate that each is similarily effective for improving endurance when the exercise regimens are comparable with respect to intensity, frequency and duration of effort (Pollock, et al, 1971; 1978). The data in Figure 10 suggest that training effectiveness is independent of mode of activity. Thus, it appears that a variety of aerobic activities can be interchanged for improving and maintaining fitness if the intensity, frequency and duration are the same.

Moderate to high level activities such as walking, jogging, swimming and cycling develop significant increases in cardiopulmonary fitness. Low level activities (sub-threshold) and intermittent sports such as bowling, golf, calesthenics, etc, are of limited value in improving fitness. Table 16 contains a summary of the energy cost of various activities.

Higdon (1977) has rated different sports and forms of exercise with respect to their ability to enhance endurance fitness. Each activity is evaluated for aerobic potential and assigned a rating code indicative of its effectiveness. Activities are rated zero to 4 stars. A four star rating is assigned to activities that provide the best route to fitness while a score of zero is reserved for activities that provide no fitness benefits. To earn a four star rating, an activity must provide a minimum of 15 aerobic points per hour, require an energy cost of at least 17.5 ml O_2/Kg·min and burn at least 500 calories per hour. A summary of Higdon's findings follows.

Walking. By definition, walking is locomotion at speeds less than 5 miles per hour. Velocities between 5 and 7 mph represent jogging, while those over 7 mph represent running. Walking is probably the least demanding of all exercises and can be engaged in by people of all ages, all body types and all levels of skill. For adults and low fit individuals, walking is the training modality most often prescribed. Most authorities recommend an initial 3 to 4 week period of walking followed by 3 to 4 weeks of walking and jogging. After 6 to 8 weeks of walking and jogging, most participants are permitted to jog continuously for specified periods of time.

FIGURE 10

EFFECT OF DIFFERENT MODES OF TRAINING ON

AEROBIC CAPACITY*

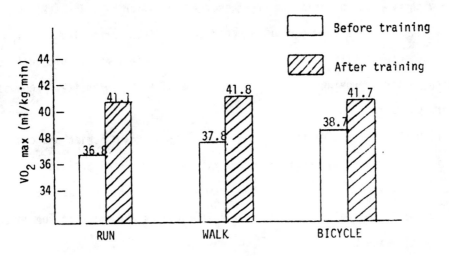

* Pollock. et al. 1978.

TABLE 16
ENERGY COST OF SELECTED ACTIVITIES

Activity	Calories/minute*
Basketball (half-court)	5.6
Bicycling (13 mph)	12.1
Calisthenics	5.6
Dancing	3.3-7.7
Football	8.9
Golf	5.0
Handball	11.0
Canoeing (4 mph)	7.9
Hiking (40 lb pack, 3 mph)	7.7
Judo, Karate	14.5
Racquetball	9.0
Rope jumping (110 rpm)	11.0

Rowing   51 str/min
            87 str/min
            97 str/min
	4.1
	7.0
	11.2

Running (5.5 - 9 mph)	12.1-17.5
Tennis	7.1
Skiing (downhill)	10.8-15.9
Squash	10.9

Swimming   Breaststroke
            Backstroke
            Crawl (55 yd/min)
	11.0
	11.5
	14.0

XBX, 5BX, Chart 1-6	9.3-18.7

* 170 pound (77 kg) person

As previously mentioned, research (Pollock, et al, 1978) comparing the effects of walking to that of jogging and cycling indicates that walking is as effective as the other two modalities for affecting changes in physical fitness. Data also indicate that walking can significantly influence body weight and body fat levels (Pollock, et al, 1971). Calculations suggest that the caloric cost of walking is approximately 90 calories per mile. This value will vary with body weight. Readers should consult Table 17 for a more precise estimate of energy cost. Additional advantages of walking include:

(1) It can be done by anyone, anytime and any place.

(2) No special equipment or clothing is required.

(3) For shy individuals, it is inconspicuous.

(4) The risk of injury is minimal.

The lone disadvantage to walking is that it is time consuming. Walkers are sometimes disturbed to discover that running is 3 to 4 times more efficient than walking. A walker (20 min/mile) will usually have to walk 30-32 minutes to achieve an energy expenditure equivalent to running one 8-minute mile. Higdon has awarded walking a 3-star rating.

Jogging-Running. Jogging, locomotion at speeds of 5 to 7 mph, and running, locomotion at speeds in excess of 7 mph, is the most efficient form of exercise. According to Cooper (1977), you can earn more aerobic points in less time by running than any other activity. The figures in Table 18 substantiate these claims. Inspection of this Table indicates that you would have to play 7 hours of golf, 50-55 minutes of tennis singles, swim 15-20 minutes or play 30 minutes of basketball to achieve the physiological stress required in running a mile in 8 to 10 minutes.

Weight conscious individuals are pleased to learn that the caloric cost of running a mile is approximately 10 calories. Since caloric cost varies somewhat with weight, readers should consult Table 19 to determine individual costs. It is important to note that the caloric cost per mile is independent of running speed.

TABLE 17
ENERGY COST OF WALKING*

Body Weight (lbs)

	100	120	140	160	180	200	220
Kcal/min	2.7	3.2	3.8	4.3	4.8	5.3	5.8
Kcal/mile	52	62	72	82	92	102	112

* 3.0 - 3.3 mph (80 - 88 m/min)

TABLE 18

AEROBIC POINT VALUE OF SELECTED ACTIVITIES*

Activity	Distance (miles)	Duration (minutes)	Aerobic Points
Basketball		25-30	4.0
Calisthenics		60	1.5
Cycling	4	12-16	4.5
Dancing (Hustle, etc.)		30	2.0
Football		40-45	4.0
Golf (24-26 holes)			4.0
Handball		25-30	4.0
Racquetball		25-30	4.0
Rope Skipping (70-90 st/min)		15	4.5
Skating		60	4.0
Swimming	.40	16-21	4.3
Volleyball		60	4.0
Tennis		60	4.5

* Cooper, 1978.

TABLE 19
ENERGY COST OF RUNNING*

	Body Weight (lbs)						
	100	120	140	160	180	200	220
Kcal/min	8.1	9.7	11.3	12.9	14.5	16.1	19.5
Kcal/mile	81	97	113	129	145	161	195

* 8-10 min/mile (160-210 m/min)

Inspection of Table 19 indicates that the caloric cost of running a 7-minute mile (17.3 calories per minute) is significantly greater than that required to run a 10-minute mile (12.5 calories/minute). The cost per mile; however, is independent of running speed. An individual running at 10-minute mile pace burns approximately 12.5 calories per minute for 10 minutes (12.5 calories/minute X 10 minutes = 125 calories) for a total cost of 125 calories. Likewise, the same individual running at 7-minute mile pace burns more calories per minute (17.3 calories/minute), but for fewer minutes (7 minutes). Thus, the total cost of the faster mile (17.3 calories/minute X 7 minutes = 121.2 calories/mile) is almost identical to that required in running at a slower pace.

Scientific study suggests that sustained aerobic activities, such as running, facilitate the metabolism of free fatty acids in the blood stream (Mole, et al, 1971; Morgan, et al, 1971). Apparently, fat metabolism is more efficient with sustained, low-moderate intensity activities such as running, cycling, etc.

Other advantages of running include:

(1) It is simple, requiring no special talent, ability or skill.

(2) It is inexpensive, requiring no special equipment, except a good pair of shoes Participants need no special facilities, club memberships, etc. Most individuals jog around the block.

(3) It is versatile, you can run in all forms of weather and in most places in the world.

(4) It is a life-time activity that can be performed by individuals of all ages.

On the negative side of the ledger, running can strain the joints of the body. Joint strain is more common if you run in small areas; run in shoes that are poorly designed, ill fitting or worn-out or if you try to run too hard or too far too soon. Research suggests that most running injuries are due to over-exertion. A study (Van Pelt, et al, 1978) of 846 participants in the 1978 Houston Marathon indicates that most frequent running injury is blisters (21%), followed in descending order by pain in the knees (18%), ankles (9%) and hips (5%).

According to Higdon (1977), running is a 4-star activity that presents a relatively low potential for injury. Sample starter programs, safe progression schedules, stretching exercises, equipment needs, environmental considerations, precautions and contraindications to exercise are presented to help the reader design a safe and effective running program.

Cycling. The data presented in Table 20 indicates that cycling can stress the cardiopulmonary system sufficiently to induce changes in aerobic fitness (Adams, 1975). Cycling at a speed of 15 mph (4:00/mile) will require an energy cost of approximately 42 ml O_2/Kg/min which is about the same as running an 8-minute mile. Cycling at an 8:00 minute mile pace (7.5 mph); however, requires only 28 ml O_2/Kg/min. Inspection of Figure 11 suggests that a cyclist riding at a given speed must travel approximately 3 miles in order to achieve the training effect derived from running 1 mile at a similar speed. Since a bicycle can travel at higher speeds, a cyclist can reduce his training time by riding at a faster velocity. The data in Figure 11 suggest that the speed of the cyclist would have to be twice as fast as that of a jogger to achieve a similar work output. The traffic congestion in most cities; however, often makes it impossible and unsafe to attempt to ride at these velocities.

Weight conscious individuals should realize that the caloric cost of cycling is approximately 50 calories per mile as compared to 120 calories per mile for jogging. Thus, the cyclist would have to travel 3 times as far to burn a similar number of calories.

While cycling is a relatively easy activity to perform, it is not without limitations. A few of the problems observed with cycling include:

(1) You must have a bicycle. Bicycles, which range in price from $80 to $800, are machines and thus breakdown, have flats and are subject to theft.

(2) Cyclists are sometimes hampered by the weather. Strong headwinds increase resistance while ice and snow render roads dangerous and/or impassable.

(3) Modern, streamlined racing bicycles are not designed for mature adults.

TABLE 20

ENERGY COST OF CYCLING*

	Speed (mph)							
	6	8	10	12	14	16	18	20
Kcal/min	1.5	3.6	5.7	7.8	9.8	11.9	14.0	16.0
Kcal/mile	15	27	34	39	42	45	47	48

* 170 lb (77 kg) individual

FIGURE 11

ENERGY COST OF RUNNING VS CYCLING

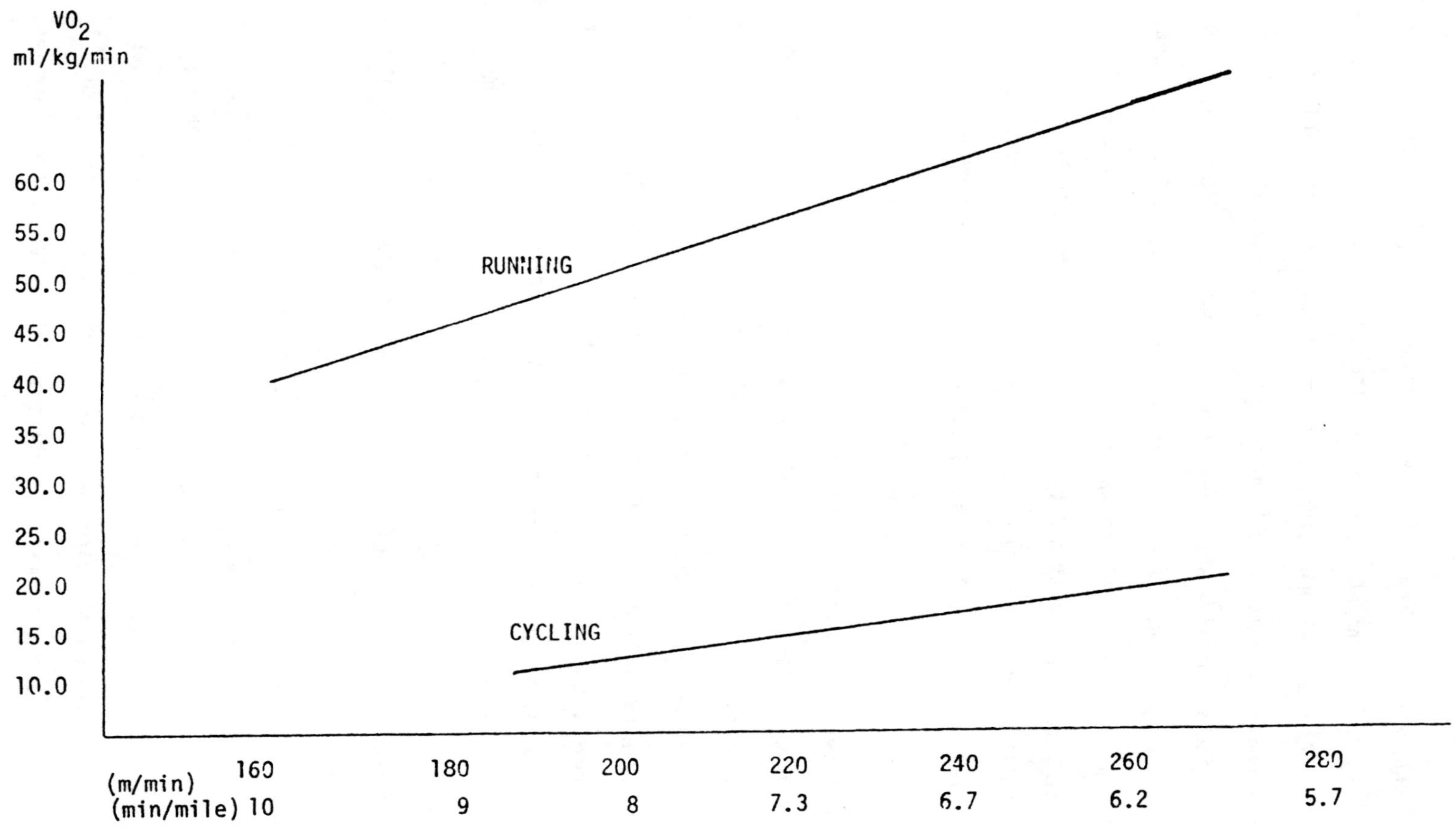

The seat, which can become extremely uncomfortable, is raised, displaces the body forward and places stress on the back and shoulders.

(4) Safety. City and residential streets are not designed to safely facilitate a steady flow of sustained, high speed cycling. Cyclists must share road space with automobiles which have a greater mass and travel at higher velocities. In a collision with an auto, only the cyclist gets hurt.

(5) Work is limited primarily to the musculature of the lower extremities.

The arm, shoulder, chest and trunk areas are relatively inactive in cycling. Higdon (1977) awards cycling a 4-star rating. However, one must consider the safety, comfort and logistics problems associated with cycling before adopting this form of aerobic training.

Swimming. Swimming is another 4-star activity with minimum potential for injury. Individuals who utilize this form of training are lap swimmers who regularly swim 400 to 800 yards. Swimming occurs in a relatively small area and thus provides the opportunity to develop a somewhat social atmosphere. Many individuals associate swimming with recreation and often view it as being more enjoyable than running. Water a warm, bouyant medium, soothes the body and tends to facilitate relaxation. Swimming exercises the total body and enhances cardiovascular and musculoskeletal (primarily arms, shoulder and legs) development. Finally, since the density of water is greater than that of fat, overweight individuals tend to float and have fewer limitations while swimming than generally encountered in running or skill activities.

Because of the tremendous variability among swimmers in style and efficiency, it is difficult to achieve a precise estimate of the energy cost of swimming. Limited research (Faulkner, 1966, 1968) on trained swimmers indicates that swimming burns approximately 300 calories per hour compared to 900 for running. Cooper (1977) awards 5 points for swimming 600 yards in 10 to 15 minutes or running 1 mile in 6 to 8 minutes. Thus, swimmers must swim approximately twice as long (minutes) to earn the same number of points as runners.

While swimming is a safe, enjoyable and effective method of training, it is not without faults. The primary requisite for swimming is a pool or appropriate body of water. For most individuals access to a pool is a minimal problem. The principle problems are:

(1) Travel to and from the facility. Research suggests that the drop-out rate among individuals who have to commute to training facilities is at least 50 percent (Harris, 1978).

(2) Weather. Unless the pool is heated and covered, adherence is extremely difficult in cold or rainy weather.

(3) Skill. In order to receive a training effect from swimming you must be able to swim continuously for 10-15 minutes. A number of individuals do not swim well enough to achieve a training threshold.

Stationary Running. Running in-place differs from ordinary running in that you do not go anywhere. The energy cost has been estimated to be approximately 400 calories per hour (6.7 calories/minute) at 80 to 90 steps per minute. A precise estimate is difficult due to variances induced by altering step height. Stationary running can be performed in-doors when the weather is bad, during travel or at times when you prefer not to run outdoors.

The principle problems with running in-place are boredom and injury. Stationary running for 8 to 10 minutes can become extremely boring. After 2 to 3 days of stationary running, most individuals find that their motivation for exercise has decreased. Some participants attempt to alleviate boredom by running in front of the TV, running to music or running through the house. Each of these solutions is temporary at best and does nothing to minimize the stresses received by the arches, ankles, knees and hips with the fall of each foot. Running within the house subjects the runner to additional torsion injuries associated with short, quick turns required to avoid furniture, pets and walls. Higdon gives stationary running 3 stars. He also indicates that boredom and musculoskeletal injury are definite problems.

Stationary Cycling. Riding an exercise bicycle (bicycle ergometer) is a safe, effective mode of training (3-star). Studies (Pollock, 1973) indicate that significant improvements can occur with cycling provided the principle of progressive resistance exercise is observed. Ergometers are safer than bicycles and enable the rider to avoid the problems associated with collisions, inclement weather and neighborhood dogs. Good ergometers, those that permit accurate assessment of rate (speed), quantity (distance) and quality (amount) of work are relatively expensive ($00-$2000). With time, most riders find stationary cycling boring and utilize TVs and radios to break the monotony. Users of stationary cycles find that training is often interrupted during travel and must seek alternative sources of exercise.

Racquetball. Racquetball is a 3-star activity with a relatively high potential for injury. The predominate injuries in racquetball are strains and sprains of lower extremities, contusions and lacerations from collisions with walls, opponents, balls and racquets. The sport is fun, easy to learn and is played with equal ability by members of both sexes. Racquetball requires strategy and finesse and is usually played in a club or social atmosphere. Equipment is relatively cheap but club membership and court fees can be expensive and limit access to facilities.

Racquetball is a new and demanding sport and has not been adequately researched. It requires approximately 10 calories per minute (600 calories/hour). Sucessful play requires that players make repeated, sudden starts and stops. This type of activity utilized carbohydrate stores and does little to metabolize fat. The accelleration-decelleration nature of the game elevates body and muscle temperature and causes participants to sweat profusely. Some individuals associate sweat with training and, unfortunately, over-estimate their level of cardiopulmonary fitness.

Some physicians are concerned that racquetball can be a hazard to the health of some participants. Since it is easy to learn, players come to the courts in relatively poor physical condition, do limited or no warm-up exercises and play with reckless abandon. The end result is a rash of sore muscles, strained backs and twisted ankles.

Older individuals and those with primary risk factors of heart disease should be cautioned about the problems associated with activities that require repeated bursts of all-out physical effort.

Handball. Handball is a sport somewhat similar to racquetball in terms of training effectiveness (2-star) and injury potential (high). It requires more upper body strength, more agility and coordination than racuqetball. In addition, one must be able to use the non-dominate hand. Like racquetball, the energy cost of this sport is related to the ability levels of the participants. Opponents of similar ability will expend more energy than those of differing ability. Since the ball is harder and hit by the hand, a handball does not travel as fast as a racquetball. Thus, handball players probably move less during competition than racquetball players.

Handball is physically a more demanding sport than racquetball. Few women participate in the game. Competition between the sexes is often biased to the male since he usually possesses more upper body strength. With the exception of contusions to the hand and dislocated or broken fingers, the injuries sustained in handball are very similar to those seen in racquetball.

Basketball. Basketball is another rapid start, sudden stop, 2-star, high risk activity. While basketball players must be strong, quick, agile and powerful, the start-stop nature of the game limits its aerobic effectiveness. The data in Table 21 indicates that 12 weeks of intercollegiate basketball was not effective in improving aerobic capacity in male players (Coleman and Kreuzer, 1974). Anaerobic power; however, did increase by approximately 6 percent. Similar observations have been reported for other collegiate males (Campbell, 1968) and for collegiate females (McArdle, et al, 1972

Some authorities estimate that basketball players burn approximately 5 calories per minute (286 calories/hour). These estimates are, in general, for collegiate athletes. The true energy cost is dependent upon the speed of the game and the intensity of individual play. One-on-one and half-court play tend to be at a slower pace and require less running. Higdon (1977) contends that shooting baskets in the backyard is not basketball, it is shooting baskets and is not aerobic.

TABLE 21

PHYSIOLOGICAL CHANGES WITH A SEASON OF
INTERCOLLEGIATE BASKETBALL*

Criterion	Preseason	Postseason	Change
Weight (lbs)	191.0	192.0	1.0
VO_2 max (ml/kg/min)	46.9	46.0	-.9
Power (ft-lbs/sec)	952.0	1016.7	64.1

* Coleman and Kreuzer (1974).

Because of the nature of the game and the fact that 10 players are functioning in a relatively small area, numerous injuries occur in basketball. Most injuries involve the ankle and knee and render the participant immobile for 7 to 10 days. Because of the difficulty in finding 10, well-conditioned individuals in a given gym at the same time, it is extremely difficult to consistently organize pick-up games that will be strenuous enough to induce cardiovascular benefits.

Other Team Sports. Most professional athletes are lean and muscular. For this reason, spectators assume that all team sports are effective "total body" conditioners. The truth is that most sports are anaerobic (Table 1) and most athletes utilize running, cycling and weight-training to develop sufficient strength and stamina to withstand the rigors of competition. Studies of professional athletes indicate that most possess average to good levels of aerobic capacity (Coleman, 1978; Parr and Wilmore, 1978; Raven, et al, 1976; Wilmore and Haskell, 1972). This observation is not surprising in light of the relatively low aerobic potential of most team sports. The data in Table 22 are presented to show the contrast between the aerobic capacity of athletes engaged in team sports and participants in endurance activities.

Tennis. Tennis is a 2-star activity in which the most frequent injuries are to the ankle, elbow and back. Most injuries occur to weekend participants and are caused by overexertion. A good game of tennis singles requires approximately 23 ml/O_2/kg/min earns 4.5 aerobic points per hour and burns approximately 7 calories per minute (420 calories/hour). Doubles and less competitive games have considerably lower energy requirements.

Tennis is a social game in which players are concerned with dress, comradery and sportsmanship. Far too many players over estimate the cardiovascular benefits of tennis. According to Cooper's standards (1977) an individual would have to play 60 minutes of tennis to earn the aerobic points given for running 1 mile. Doubles players would have to play for 2 hours.

Professional players appear trim, well-conditioned and capable of sustained

TABLE 22

AEROBIC CAPACITY OF MALE PARTICIPANTS IN
SELECTED ATHLETIC EVENTS

Activity	No.	Age (yrs)	Height (in)	Weight (lb)	VO_2 max ml/min	ml/kg/min	Reference
Baseball (NL)	20	25.9	73.1	188.8	4702	54.8	Coleman (1977)
Basketball (NCAA)	9	19.8	75.3	192.3	4099	46.9	Coleman and Kreuzer (1974)
Basketball (NBA)	34	25.5	79.1	212.5	4400	45.9	Parr, et al (1978)
Football (NFL)							Wilmore, et al (1976)
Def. Backs	26	24.5	71.9	186.6	4500	53.1	
Off. Backs	40	24.7	73.4	199.5	4700	52.2	
Wide Receivers	40	24.7	73.4	199.5	4700	52.2	
Linebackers	28	24.2	74.3	224.8	5300	52.1	
Off. Linemen	38	24.7	76.0	247.7	5600	49.9	
Tight Ends	38	24.7	76.0	247.7	5600	49.9	
Def. Linemen	32	25.7	75.7	257.6	5300	44.9	
Quarterback	16	24.1	84.1	198.2	4500	49.0	
Kickers	16	24.1	84.1	198.2	4500	49.0	
Soccer (NASL)	18	26.0	69.3	166.1	4409	58.4	Raven, et al (1976)
Track (AAU/NCAA)							
Elite Distance Runner	14	26.2	70.4	140.6	4946	77.4	Costill, et al (1976
Discus Throwers	7	28.3	73.3	230.3	4900	47.5	Fahey, et al
Shot Putters	5	27.0	74.1	247.5	4800	42.6	(1975)
Weightlifters (Olympics)	11	25.3	69.7	194.0	4500	50.7	

submaximal effort for 2 to 3 hours at a time. What weekend participants often fail to realize, is that the ability to maintain tennis play is influenced by regular conditioning programs (running, strength training, etc). Professional players are in shape to play tennis because of specific conditioning activities, not vice-versa.

Golf. Most authorities agree that golf is a safe, low level (1-star) social activity. Cooper (1977) gives 1.5 points for 9 holes. The energy cost of pulling a golf cart is approximately 12 ml O_2/Kg/min, the same as required in pitching horseshoes. Riding an electric cart costs approximately 9 ml/Kg/min. Research suggests that one hour of golf will burn 223 calories, approximately the same as used in running 16 minutes. Thus, golf is an expensive sport that requires expensive facilities and equipment and yields very little physiological benefit. The primary benefits of golf tend to be social and recreational.

Weight Lifting. A review of Chapter 2 indicates that weight training is an anaerobic activity and, therefore, one should not expect significant physiological changes. A few weight-lifters contend that circuit training, i.e., performing numerous sub-maximal repetitions at 10 or more stations, will elevate the heart rate and enhance endurance fitness. Recent investigations indicate that this assumption is false. Gettman, et al (1978), compared the effects of circuit weight training (CWT) to running. Eleven adult males trained for 30 minutes per day, 3 times per week. Subjects in the CWT program performed 2 sets of 10 exercises on a Universal Gym Apparatus. Fifteen repetitions with a weight equal to 50 percent of the 1-RM were performed at each station. Subjects were allowed 20-25 seconds of rest between exercises. CWT time was progressively decreased throughout the study, i.e., subjects were required to complete the prescribed number of repetitions/lifts in less time. Likewise, the weight load lifted was also increased at periodic intervals.

Members of the running group exercised at 85 percent of maximum heart rate for 23 to 27 minutes per workout. Participants in the CWT group exercised at a heart rate of 79-84 percent of maximum. Analysis of results indicated that the runners observed a 13 percent increase in aerobic capacity while the CWT group recorded only a 3 percent gain.

Wilmore, et al (1978) measured the energy cost of CWT in 20 adult males and 20 adult females. Subjects performed 3 circuits (10 stations per circuit) using a work (30-sec) to rest (15-sec) ratio of 2:1 and a total exercise time of 22.5 minutes. Analysis of data indicated that the average energy expenditure for males was 9 calories/ minute (540 calories/hour). For females this value was 6.1 calories/minute (386 calories/hour).

Weight conscious individuals would have to perform approximately 9 circuits per hour to achieve a caloric expenditude equivalent to running 2 to 3 miles in 16 to 24 minutes. Most weightlifters use heavier weights and lift them at slower rates than those utilized in the aforementioned studies. Therefore, one should expect a lower energy cost with traditional strength training procedures than observed with CWT.

Weight training must be accepted for what it is, an excellent means of increasing muscle size and strength. Runners must utilize some form of strength training to increase muscular strength. Weightlifters must engage in some form of aerobic exercise to enhance endurance fitness.

Calisthenics. Most authorities suggest that calisthenics are best used as a warm-up exercise before running or engaging in competitive sports. The caloric cost of calisthenics varies with the type of activity used, rate of movement, range of movement and weight of the participant. Estimates indicate that the typical adult should burn approximately 360 calories per hour performing calisthenics. Cooper awards only 1.5 points for 60 minutes of calisthenics. Thus, one would have to exercise for approximately 2.5 hours to achieve the aerobic points attributable to running 1 mile.

Dancing. Until recently, most dancing was social and was not considered to have physiological benefits. Recent interest in aerobic dance and disco have led investigators to examine the energy cost of dancing. Studies of aerobic dance indicate that dancing can have a positive effect on endurance fitness. Foster (1975) collected expired air on female participants in an aerobic dance workshop and found

the energy cost of a typical dance routine to be approximately 33.6 ml O_2/Kg/min.
Similar observations have been reported by Weber (1974) who found that the energy cost
30 minutes of high intensity aerobic dancing with 5, 45-second rest breaks was
equivalent to 30 minutes of continuous jogging at 5.5 mph. In a study of 31 college
women enrolled in an aerobic dance class, Mass (1975) found that dancing 30 to 40
minutes per day, 2 times per week for 12 weeks significantly increased aerobic capacity
In addition to being an effective training method, dancing for most individuals is
fun and mentally relaxing. Individuals who become bored with jogging, stationary
running, etc, often find dancing a refreshing and exciting form of training.

Maintenance of Training.

An important consideration of any training procedure is how to effectively maintain the benefits gained from training. Research suggests that most physiological
changes, e.g., heart rate, VO_2 max, strength, etc, decrease with inactivity. Data
suggest that the rate of loss is, in general, proportional to the rate of gain. That
is, changes produced over several months or years are lost more slowly than those
gained over the course of a few weeks.

Studies (Hettinger, 1961; Stamford, 1978) on muscular strength indicate that
subjects who train regularly for 6 to 12 months and then cease training loose approximately 50 percent of their strength gain within 3 months and almost 100 percent within
one year. Similar observations have been reported for college and professional
athletes (Coleman, 1970; 1978; Campbell, 1967). Guess (1967) trained varsity football
players at the University of Texas for approximately 5 months. Upon completion of the
training program, the squad was divided into 2 groups. Group one participated in all
practices, games and scrimmages for 12 weeks. Group two had the same activity pattern
as Group one with one exception; they participated in strength training activities
two times per week. Comparison of post-season data indicated that participation in
games, scrimmages and practice sessions was ineffective for maintaining muscular
strength. Subjects who trained twice per week; however, were able to maintain a

significant percentage of previously developed muscular strength. Similar observations were made by Coleman (1978) among major league baseball players. Athletes who trained 3 times per week during the off-seasons and 2 times per week during the season were significantly stronger after 162 games than those who did not train during the season. These findings are consistent with those of Darden (1977) who suggests that high levels of muscular size and strength start to decrease after approximately 96 hours (4 days). Individuals who want to maintain strength should train at least every 4 days i.e., twice per week.

Changes in aerobic capacity with de-training tend to parallel those observed for msucular strength, i.e., (1) losses occur with inactivity and (2) the rate of loss is proportional to the rate of gain. Pedersen and Jorgensen (1978) studied adult females during 7 weeks of training and 7 weeks of de-training. Subjects who ceased training returned to pre-training values (VO_2 max within 7 weeks of cessation of training. Fringer and Stull (1974) trained and de-trained 44 college women on a bicycle ergometer. After 10 weeks of training, subjects were randomly assigned to one of two experimental groups. Group one ceased exercise for 5 weeks and Group two did not train for 10 weeks. When re-tested, subjects in Group one had lost approximately 68 percent of the gains in aerobic capacity within 5 weeks of cessation of training. Subjects in Group two lost 100 percent of the training induced gains after 10 weeks of inactivity.

Similar results were observed by Brynteson (1969), Cureton and Phillips (1964), Fordy (1969) and Drinkwater and Horvath (1972). The findings of Drinkwater and Horvath (1972) are especially interesting. They trained 7 teenage female track athletes for approximately 3 months, tested them for aerobic capacity, ceased formal training for 3 months and then re-tested the athletes. Results indicated that, following 3 months of de-training, the subjects had regressed to pre-training values. These results are interesting because the girls were not inactive during the de-training phase. Each was enrolled in required physical education classes such as field hockey, basketball, tennis and baseball. Apparently, these sports activities were insufficient stimuli to maintain a significant amount of the gains in aerobic capacity associated with running.

Daniels (1975) suggest that losses in aerobic capacity with inactivity are influenced by the duration of previous training. He cites that data in Table 23 as proof that rate of loss is proportional to rate of gain. The data in this Table represents a lonitudinal study of former world record holder Jim Ryun. Prior to the 1968 Olympic Games, Ryun had a VO_2 max of 79.5 ml O_2/Kg/min. After one year of inactivity (no training), his max had decreased by 18 percent to 65.0 ml O_2/Kg/min. Further analysis of metabolic data; however, indicated that his absolute VO_2 max (ml O_2/min) had decreased only 7 percent (-420 ml/min) while his body weight had increased by 9.5 Kg (+13 percent). Thus, the decrement in relative VO_2 max(ml O_2/Kg/min) was due primarily to an increase in body weight, not a reduction in physiological efficiency. Similar observations in well conditioned athletes suggest that gains obtained over years of training are affected less by periods of inactivity than those obtained quickly.

It must be emphasized, that the aforementioned findings were observed on individuals who had trained continuously for years. Individuals who participate in "one-shot" programs such as those utilized in the military (basic training) and similar agencies will find that participation in 6 week to 6 month structured programs will not ensure fitness for life. Recent studies of police and military personnel who had completed 4 to 6 months of rigorous recruit training indicated the need for physical fitness maintenance activities (Stamford, et al, 1978). When participants were re-examined after 6 to 12 months of active duty, the data revealed a significant decrease in aerobic fitness and muscular strength and a significant increase in body fat.

Scientific data suggest that the effort required to maintain fitness is less than that required to gain fitness (Mathews and Fox, 1976). Studies indicate that a significant portion of training induced changes in muscular strength and endurance fitness can be maintained with submaximal efforts performed as few as two times per

TABLE 23

CHANGES IN AEROBIC CAPACITY WITH

DE-TRAINING: JIM RYUN, A CASE STUDY*

Year	1967	1968	1968	1970	1970	1970	1970	1971	1972
Age	20	21	21	23	23	23	23	24	25
% Fat				10.1	9.0	8.1	7.0		6.7
Wt (kg)	73.0	73.0	72.5	82.0	79.5	77.2	76.2	73.2	75.3
max VO_2 (ml/min)	5910	5650	5755	5335	5595	5600	5400	5511	5900
(ml/Kg/min)	81.0	77.5	79.5	65.0	70.4	72.5	74.0	75.2	78.3
max VE (L/BTPS)	190	184	180	185	184	185	180	185	198
Rest HR	72			76		76	64		
Max HR	180	160		180	180	176	176	175	

* Daniels. 1976.

week.

Cooper (1977) advocates that individuals utilize endurance activities such as walking, joggin, cycling or swimming to establish a sound aerobic base. The criteria for achieving a sound aerobic base for men under 30 years of age is a VO_2 max of 42 ml O_2/Kg/min. For women, this value is 36 ml O_2/Kg/min. Since VO_2 max decreases with age, the guidelines have been adjusted for age differences and are presented in Table 6. Once the aerobic base is established and a sufficient level of fitness is attained, he recommends that participants utilize a variety of aerobic activities and/or sports to maintain cardiopulmonary fitness. Numerous activities have been classified with respect to their ability to tax the cardiopulmonary system and a point system has been assigned relative to their effectiveness. For example, jogging 1 mile in 8 to 10 minutes will earn the participant 4 aerobic points. Cycling 3 miles in less than 9 minutes will earn the participant 4.5 points, as will swimming 550 yards in 9 to 14 minutes. Sports such as golf, tennis, racquetball, and basketball are less aerobic in nature and must be performed for longer periods of time in order to yield substantial aerobic points.

According to Cooper (1977), aerobic fitness can be maintained if an individual is sufficiently active to earn 30 points per week. Women are urged to earn 24 points Any combination of activities is permitted so long as the end result is a total of 30 or 24 points per week for men and women, respectively. Popular combinations are presented in Table 24. The data in Table 25 is presented as proof that a relationship exists between endurance fitness level and aerobic points earned per week (Cooper, 1977) Inspection of this Table indicates that at least 30 points per week are necessary to achieve a fitness classification of "good."

While the primary emphasis of Cooper's earlier texts has been endurance fitness, more recent work (1980) has emphasized the importance of muscular strength. Members of the Aerobics Activity Center in Dallas, Texas are encouraged to utilize a daily conditioning program consisting of the following 4 stages:

(1) <u>Warm-up</u>. Participants stretch and perform light calisthenics for 2 to 5

TABLE 24

ALTERNATIVE AEROBIC TRAINING ACTIVITIES

Activity	Distance (miles)	Time (min:sec)	Freq/week	Points	Points/wk	Total
Jogging and		8:01-10:00	3	4.0	12	32.0
Racquetball	1.00	55:00-59:59	2	10.0	20	
Swimming and		11:16-15:01	4	3.0	12	25.7
Tennis Singles	.25	60:00	3	4.5	13.5	
Jogging,	2.00	16:01-20:00	1	9.0	9	31.4
Cycling,	(20 mph)	14:00	2	3.0	6	
Swimming and	.25	11:16-15:01	1	3.0	3	
Tennis Singles		90:00	2	6.7	13.4	

TABLE 25

RELATIONSHIP BETWEEN AEROBIC CAPACITY
AND AEROBIC POINT PERFORMANCE*

Fitness Category	Number	Points/Week
Very Poor	16	17.1
Poor	44	17.2
Fair	86	18.5
Good	226	34.6
Excellent	202	50.0

* Cooper (1977); 574 males, mean age 44.5 years; first visit

minutes to increase general circulation and prepare the musculo-skeletal system for additional work.

(2) Aerobics. Participants engage in walking, running, cycling, swimming or approved sports. The minimum duration of this period is approximately 20 minutes.

(3) Cool Down. Participants taper-off by walking, jogging and/or stretching slowly for approximately 5 minutes in order to allow the muscles to help restore central circulation. An abrupt cessation of exercise allows the peripheral blood flow developed during activity to pool in the extremities and may precipitate fainting. A reasonable index of recovery is a heart rate of less than 120 bpm after 5 minutes.

(4) Strength Training. Weight training, calisthenics, etc, designed to enhance muscle tone and strength are performed for 10-15 minutes after the cool down period.

Training, Age and Initial Status. Chronological age and starting level of fitness are important determinants of training potential. In general, the lower the age and the lower the initial level of fitness the greater the potential for improvement (Figure 12). This does not imply that a person with a low level of fitness has a greater chance to attain a higher terminal value, but relates to the potential for percentage increase. While the figures of 10 to 20 percent are often cited as the average range of improvement following endurance fitness training, actual values may vary somewhat with the age and initial capacity of the participant. Saltin, et al (1968) trained 5 "normal" subjects who had been confined to bed for 20 days, for 50 days and observed a 33 percent increase in VO_2 max. Similar observations have been reported for others whose capacity had declined because of health and/or environmental restrictions (Hollman, 1965; Jones, et al, 1962; Ekblom, et al, 1968).

The fact that the potential for improvement decreases somewhat with age does not indicate that age is a barrier to training (Bary, 1966; Becklace, 1965; Benestal, 1965)

FIGURE 12
AGE AND TRAINABILITY*

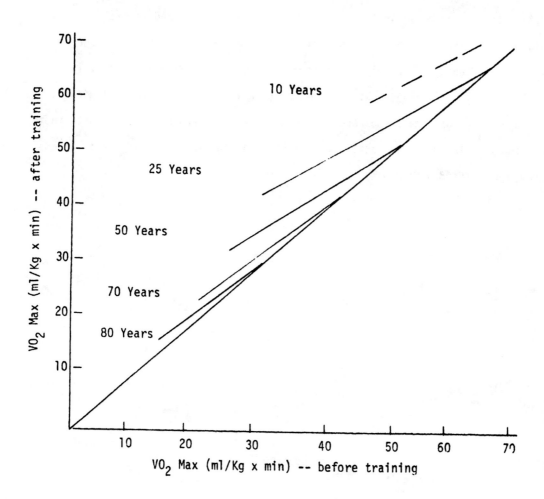

*Daniels (1977)

Studies involving adults 35 to 60 years of age indicate that most can improve aerobic capacity by 10 to 20 percent with regular training (Hollmann, 1965; Pollock, et al, 1973). Similar results have been observed for older adults and several reports have been published to indicate that males and females over 60 years of age have the potential to train and run distances from 1 to 26 miles (Balke and Clark, 1961; Cureton, 1964; Dill, 1965). Wilmore, et al (1974), studied the physiological characteristics of 3 male endurance athletes 72 to 74 years of age. Results indicated that individuals who remain active can maintain a high level of endurance fitness through at least 8 decades.

CHAPTER 5
Body Composition

The American public is pre-occupied with body weight. Results of the November
1979 Harris Poll indicate that the number 1 leisure-time activity in America is
eating, followed closely by watching TV and, I assume, eating while watching TV.
The typical adult goes on and off approximately 1.4 diets per year. Some figures
suggest that approximately 25 to 45 percent of the population is overweight (Hofmann,
1978). During the past decade we have witnessed a tremendous increase in the volume
of diet books published each year. Schanche (1974) contends that several million
diet books are published each year and sales records indicate that they are being consumed by the public in record number. Three of the current 10 best selling, non-
fiction books are diet books. Since the invention of the printing press, only 2
books, the Bible and dictionaries, have sold more volumes than diet books.
Why are Americans obsessed with diet? Diet is the major determinant of body weight an
excess weight has been linked to a variety of chronic degenerative diseases. Overweight individuals, in general:

1) have more gallbladder disease

2) are more prone to hypertension

3) have a higher incidence of atherosclerosis

4) suffer more congestive heart failure

5) experience more digestive disease

6) have more kidney disease

7) are more prone to develop diabetes and

8) have a shorter life expectancy

In addition, individuals who are overweight have a greater incidence of respiratory
infections, miss more days of work, have a lower tolerance to exercise and are more
lethargic due to specific biochemical changes associated with increased body fat, and
thus are less productive professionally and socially (Pollock, et al, 1977; Cooper, 19

Finally, there is a definite social stigma to obesity in our society which tends to discriminate against overweight individials and thus restricts professional growth, impairs social opportunities and lowers self-esteem. Research at Northwestern University Memorial Hospital in Chicago indicates that employers often view fat people as second-class citizens and discriminate against them in hiring and promotional practices. For example, the employment rate among fat people in Chicago is 14 percent below average. Body fat can also effect earning power. Studies suggest that, among executives, 35 percent of those in the $10,000 to $20,000 salary range are more than 10 pounds overweight. In the $25,000 to $50,000 salary range, less than 10 percent are overweight. Individuals and employers are discovering that a robust figure is no longer a sign of success. Professional advantages and social opportunities are being extended more and more to trim individuals.

As a nation, we have begun to realize the potential problems associated with excess body weight. Unfortunately, too many are incapable of exercising the self-restraint necessary to safely reduce weight. Thus, we migrate from diet to diet seeking a fast, easy method of loosing weight.

The relationship between weight and body fat. While most people are concerned with body weight, weight alone is not the cause of most of our health and appearance problems. The culprit is body fat, not weight. Insurance statistics indicate that we are overweight, i.e., too heavy for our height. Anthropometric data suggest that we are too fat. Statistics indicate that 30 percent of adult males, 40 percent of adult females and 20 percent of American teen-agers have enough body fat to be classified as being obese. Obesity is determined by calculating body fat and comparing the figure obtained to established standards.

Body fatness is determined through a process known as body composition assessment (Behnke and Wilmore, 1974). A number of relatively simple indirect techniques have been developed to estimate the body's composition in the living human. The majoriety of these techniques fractionate the body into two components, lean body weight and fat weight. Lean body weight includes muscle, bone, connecutive tissue, organ and fluid weight, i.e., that portion of the body that is not fat. The remaining portion of body weight is body fat. Total body fat exists in two basic sites. Essential fat is stored in the marrow of the bones and in organs such as the heart, lungs, liver, spleen, kidneys, intestines, spinal cord and brain. Storage fat, the fat that accumulates in the adipose tissue, consists of fatty tissues that protect the various organs from trauma and the subcutaneous fat deposited beneath the skin. It is this subcutaneous fat that gives us a rounded appearance, tugs on the pelvis and produces structural changes in the neck, shoulders and pelvis.

The size of the storage depot of fat can vary considerably with age, sex, fitness and nutritional status. Experiments suggest that the lower limit of fatness in males is approximately 3 to 4 percent of body weight (Katch and McArdle, 1977). In women, this limit appears to be approximately 10 to 12 percent. Studies of female distance runners and women suffering from anorexia nervosa indicate that the reproduct system ceases to function properly when body fat levels become too low. Drinkwater, et (1978) observed that menstrual flow ceased in female runners when body fat fell below 10 percent.

What causes obesity? Obesity occurs when an individual's diet produces more fuel than is needed to maintain body functions and meet the requirements of daily activities. Excess food is stored as fatty tissue throughout the body and gradually increases with age and inactivity. From this definition, it would appear that weight (fat) control is simply a matter of eating fewer calories than needed and burning the excess fat as fuel to meet daily energy needs. While dietary restriction is essential for weight control, it is not the sole solution. Several interrelated factors usually exist in cases of obesity.

Obesity runs in families. Specific causes may be both genetic and environmental. In studies of children, Mayer (1968) found that 10 percent of the children of normal weight parents were obese. The proportions rose to 40 percent if one parent was obese and to 80 percent if both parents were obese. The tendency to be fat may be related to heredity or could be attributable, in part, to parental attitude toward food and between meal snacks. Research also suggests that fat children tend to become fat adults. A study in Maryland indicated that 86 percent of overweight boys became overweight adults as compared to 42 percent of the boys of average weight. Among females 80 percent of overweight girls became overweight women as compared to only 18 percent of girls of average weight.

Reducing Body Fat. Lack of exercise has also been shown to be positively related to body fatness. The figures in Table 24 illustrate the fact that individuals can become fatter without increasing body weight. With age and inactivity, muscles atrophy. If diet is held constant, this muscle mass is replaced by fat and total body fat increases despite a maintenance of body weight.

Likewise, individuals who rely on diet alone to reduce body fatness loose less fat than those who combine diet and exercise (Oscai, et al, 1974; Pollock, 1977; Wilmore, 1977). With dietary restriction individuals tend to loose both fat and lean body weight. Studies of fasting adults indicated that the ratio of fat to lean weight loss was approximately 50:50. Upon cessation of the fast, weight was regained. Unfortunately, because of the sedentary nature of the dieters, both the lean body weight and fat weight that had been lost were replaced by fat. Thus, the individuals became fatter despite the fact that they had been on a diet and had not increased body weight above the pre-diet values.

The most effective approach to weight control is diet and exercise. With exercise you elevate the metabolic rate, burn calories as you exercise and burn additional calories after exercise as the metabolic rate gradually returns to normal values over time. The magnitude of this residual, post-exercise increase in metabolic rate has not been thoroughly examined. Preliminary data suggest that it is significant and is influenced by the intensity and duration of the exercise. Following prolonged, near-maximal exercise, metabolism can remain elevated up to 12 to 24 hours. In increased oxygen consumption of only 100 ml/ minute (1.4 ml/kg/min for a 70 kg subject) will amount to approximately .5 calories per minute or 30 calories per hour. If metabolism remains elevated for 10 hours, an additional 300 calories would be expended, the equivalent of running approximately 3 to 3.5 miles. An individual exercising at this level five times per week would expend 1500 calories, approximately .4 pounds, in one week just from the recovery period alone.

Individuals who utilize exercise and/or diet plus exercise sometimes observe that total body weight does not decrease significantly. This observation is more prevalent in individuals who are only 5 to 10 pounds overweight. With exercise you increase muscle mass as you reduce body fat. Since the density of muscle is greater than that of fat, changes do not necessarily show-up on the scales. What does occur is an increase in lean weight, a reduction in relative body fat, decreases in subcutaneous skinfolds and slight to moderate increases in muscle girth. Runners usually note a reduction in the circumference of the waist and hips and a firmness in the muscles of the buttocks, thighs and calves. Weight lifters and swimmers also observe an increase in the size and tone of the muscles of the upper extremities.

Diets. While a major segment of society is concerned with losing body weight, most of us are time-oriented and expect changes to occur immediately. Unfortunately, weight loss, like weight gain, is a slow process. A number of individuals read that running burns approximately 100 calories per mile. They also see that one pound of fat equals about 3500 calories. Simple arithmetic indicates that 35 miles must be run to loose 1 pound of fat. This revelation is extremely distressing to most over-weight, out od shape adults. If you can not run one block, you tend to ignore the fact that exercise increases leaness, reduces blood lipids, enhances cardiopulmona efficiency, increases muscle tone and improves endurance. Your immediate problem is that you are too fat and you want a quick, effective method to lose weight. Too often, these individuals turn to fad diets that promise fast, effortless results and they turn to them in record numbers. Despite scientific claims to the contrary, we spend approximately 10 billion dollars each year on fads ranging from diet books to rubber suits. Why do we ignore expert opinion, spend our money and jeopardize our health? We are a society convinced by science and technology that for each and every problem, medical, physical, mental or social, there exists some product that we can use, injest, inhale, inject, rub-on or smoke that will alleviate the problem with minimum effort or discomfort. We are overly optimistic when it comes to personal health and safety and eternally searching for a "miracle cure" or "magic pill" that will alleviate symptoms and restore health and vitality.

For this reason, we are quick to try every new, quick-loss diet that we come across Dieting, especially crash-dieting, is in vogue. Everyone knows that you can lose 6 to 8 pounds per week with a good crash diet. But where does this weight loss come from? Several studies have reported that substantial weight losses will occur with crash dieting (500 calories/day or less). However, 60 percent of the loss comes from the body's lean weight and less than 40 percent comes from fat weight. Much of the lean weight lost is in the form of water. Many crash diets require a severe restriction of carbohydrate intake. As a result, the body's stores of carbohydrate become depleted. The body's capacity for stored carbohydrate is approximately 800 grams. Each gram is in turn stored with 3 grams of water. Therefore, depletion of carbohydrate supplies results in the loss lf 1.75 pounds (800 grams) of carbohydrates, the body's most efficient source of energy, and 5 pounds (2400 grams) of water. Thus, the rapid reduction in body weight that occurs during the first week of low carbohydrate dieting is primarily water.

Fasting. It is physiologically impossible to lose more than 4 pounds of fat per week, even if you go on a starvation diet. Assuming that one pound of fat is equal to 3500 calories, an individual with a caloric requirement of 2500 calories per day would loose .7 pounds of fat per day (2500÷3500) and 4.9 pounds of fat per week (.7 pounds X 7 days) if he went on a complete fast. Unfortunately, since he consumed no food, that portion of the metabolic rate associated with assimilation, digestion and distribution of food (specific dynamic action of food) is not active which reduces metabolic rate by 20 to 25 percent. A 20 percent reduction in metabolism would reduce the daily caloric deficit to 200 calories per day (2500 calories X 80%). A 2000 calorie deficit would produce a weight loss of approximately .57 pounds of fat per day. The total loss per week would be only 4 pounds of fat (.57 pounds X 7 days). Very few individuals are able to tolerate the physical and emotional stress associated with this method of weight control.

The more sensible approach is diet and exercise. Elimination of one slice of buttered bread from the diet each day will result in a weight loss of 10 pounds per year (100 calories/day X 365 days). Combined with 20 to 30 minutes of jogging 3 times per week, this approach would result in a total weight loss of 25 to 30 pounds per year. Weight losses achieved this way seem to be more permanent. The information depicted in the Appendix illustrates the caloric value of various popular "fast-foods" sold in America. In addition, figures are presented that estimate the number of minutes that you would have to run in order to negate the caloric value of these foods This information is presented as an aid for individuals who wish to control caloric intake.

Exercise and Weight Reduction. If one accepts the fact that exercise will help control body weight, the next logical questions are: (1) What exercises are best; and (2) How much exercise do I need? The answer to the first question is aerobic exercise. Weight loss is determined by calories burned. The longer you engage in an activity, the more calories burned. Low to moderate intensity, steady state, aerobic activities can be sustained for extended periods of time and yield the best potential for caloric expenditure.

Research suggests that for effective weight loss, exercises must be performed at least 3 times per week (Pollock, et al, 1978). The greater the frequency, intensity and duration of training, the greater the weight loss. Weight loss can be enhanced if you will utilize a high-nutritious low-fat diet and restrict caloric intake by 200 to 500 calories per day. A safe weight reduction goal is no more than 2 pounds per week. A more realistic approach is approximately 1 pound per week. At least one investigator (Pollock, 1973) has indicated that middle-aged males who expend at least 400 calories per day can maintain ideal body weight without counting calories.

Dieters should consume at least 3 meals per day, including breakfast. Skipping meals results in over-indulgence at subsequent meals. Research in animals (Nisbett, 1972) has demonstrated that, given the same number of total calories, the animals that eat their food in 1 to 2 hours gain more weight than those that are required to spread their ration throughout the day.

A few individuals mistakenly believe that exercise will stimulate the appetite to such an extent that voluntary food intake will be increased. Mayer (1968) observed that the appetite in animals decreased following exercise continued for periods up to one hour. Similar results (Bray, 1969) on humans suggest that exercise might be a mild appetite suppressant. The precise cause of appetite suppression is not known, but some authorities attribute it to increased catecholamine levels which accompany sustained activity.

Spot Exercises. Many individuals are deceived by the false advertising claims proported by manufacturers of certain exercise-weight-loss apparatus. For example, spot reduction, a technique practiced by more than a few questionable health spas, is totally without scientific merit. Fat is lost from all areas in which fat is stored in the body. Fat is mobilized from those areas of greatest concentration and is not localized to the area being exercised. The significant reductions in waist girth following sit-ups is not the result of total or localized fat. These changes in girth are attributable to the strengthening of the abdominal musculature which pulls the abdominal components back into their normal position. Atrophy of abdominal muscles permits the abdominal contents to spill-out and results in a "pot belly" figure. Strengthening these muscles pulls everything into place with little or no effect on abdominal fat. Specific examples of effective abdominal exercises are presented in Chapter 7 and 8.

What About Exercising in Sweat Suits or Rubber Suits? This practice is without merit and is an extremely hazardous health practice. The weight loss following such practice is primarily water. These losses are temporary, dehydrate the participant, compromise the kidney and general cardiovascular system and are potentially danger-ous. Losses of 2 to 4 percent of total body weight severly impair physical performance

How do you Determine Ideal Body Weight? Over the years, numerous techniques for determining body fatness have evolved. For years, age related height-weight tables have been used to determine ideal body weight. Status was determined by comparing body weight to standards established for individuals of similar age, sex and height. Individuals who were 7 to 10 percent below the average for their respective population were considered to be undernourished. Those 15 to 20 percent above average were classified as being obese. Recent research has cast considerable doubt on the validity of this procedure. Height-weight assessment has been criticized because body build, skeletal size, muscle mass and body fat are not considered in the final assessment. Two individuals of the same age, height and weight, one muscular with little fat, the other weak with generous amounts of adipose tissue would receive the same classification according to most tables.

The figures in the following example illustrate the difficulty in assessing nutritional status in lean, compromise individual on the basis of height-weight tables. A popular major league baseball player was measured and observed to be of large frame, 74 inches tall and 220 pounds in weight. According to tables, this player exceeded his ideal weight (184 pounds) by 36 pounds. When evaluated for body compo-sition, the player was determined to be only 9 percent fat and possessed 200 pounds of lean weight and 20 pounds of fat weight. In order to reach the target weight identified from the tables, this player would have to eliminate all body fat and loose 16 pounds of lean weight. Such an approach would be impossible and a needless detriment to his health and athletic performance and illustrates the fallacy of attempting to determine ideal weight without adequate knowledge of body build, lean weight and fat weight.

Several accurate techniques exist for assessing body fatness. One widely used method uses hydrostatic weighing to determine body volume. This procedure measures an individual's weight while dry and while totally submerged under water. The loss of weight in water (dry weight-underwater weight) is equivalent to the volume of the body (Archimedes). The obtained value is corrected for the volume of air trapped in the lungs and water density. Body density is then determined by dividing dry weight by the corrected body volume (density = dry weight ÷ body volume). Equations are used to convert body density to relative or % body fat (% fat = (495 ÷ density) 450). Once relative fat is determined, fat weight is calculated as the product of total body weight and relative body fat. Lean weight is the difference between total body weight and fat weight.

A simpler, more widely used, but less accurate method of assessing body composition consists of measuring the thickness of various subcutaneous fat deposits. Since approximately 50 percent of the body's total fat content is located in the tissues beneath the skin, assessment of subcutaneous thickness will provide a reliable estimate of body fatness. The procedure consists of grasping, with the thumb and forefinger, a fold of skin and subcutaneous fat away from the underlying muscular tissue. The thickness of this double layer of tissue is then measured with a skin-fold caliper (micrometer). Several sites are measured according to standardized procedures, the results are entered into specific regression equations and relative body fat is calculated. Since subcutaneous fat tends to vary with age and sex, equations have been developed for specific populations. Specific procedures for assessing body composition by skinfold analysis are presented in Chapter 8. Once relative fat (% fat) is determined, tables can be consulted and an individual can be classified with respect to fatness-leaness. Sample classification indicies are presented in Table 26.

TABLE 26
BODY FAT CLASSIFICATION

CLASSIFICATION	MEN	WOMEN
Excellent	0.6.3	0 - 8.0
Very Good	6.4 - 7.2	8.1 - 11.0
Above Average	7.3 - 9.0	11.1 - 14.0
Average	9.1 - 12.2	14.1 - 17.0
Below Average	12.3 - 13.1	17.1 - 19.0
Poor	13.2 - 19.9	19.1 - 24.0
Very Poor	20 +	25 +

CHAPTER 6
Flexibility

Flexibility is the ability to bend, twist and stretch. Anthropologists and therapists assess flexibility with the use of gonimeters and/or flexometer and define it as the range of possible movement in a specific joint or series of joints. Physical educators and trainers determine flexibility from a series of performance measurements such as the sit-and-reach and trunk extension tests. These tests assess regional flexibility and are less precise than the aforementioned clinical techniques. While it is possible to make comparisons among individuals on the basis of performance tests, these tests are better used as screening and motivational instruments. Since no allowances are made for physical stature, it is possible for a relatively inflexible individual with long upper body and arms and short legs to score as well or better than a more flexible colleagues with shorter limbs. Also, it should be noted that flexibility is specific to a given joint or combination of joints. An individual is composed of a series of joints, some of which may be unusually flexible, some inflexible and some average. These tests should be reserved for determining initial status and evaluating progress. Generalizations about the total flexibility of individuals should be avoided.

Limitations to Flexibility. Flexibility varies from individual to individual and from joint to joint within a given individual. Maximal flexibility within a joint may be limited by mechanical factors and/or elasticity of soft tissue structures. Mechanical factors usually include normal bony structures such as those found in the elbow and knee joints. Such barriers are sometimes found in heavily muscled individuals in whom range of motion is limited by the bulk of the intervening muscle. Similar barriers are also observed in extremely obese individuals who often find that intervening layers of fat impede flexibility.

In joints such as the ankle and hip joint, the limitations to motion are usually imposed by soft tissues such as skeletal muscle and its fascial sheaths, connecutive tissue (tendons, ligaments and joint capsules) and skin. In a study designed to indentify the primary deterents to joint movement in animals, Johns and Wright (1962) observed that muscles, joint capsules and tendons were the most important factors in limiting free movement. In humans, resistance is thought to be centered in the fascial sheath that covers the muscle.

Importance of Flexibility. Joint flexibility is important for a variety of reasons. The most important reasons are concerned with posture, appearance and musculoskeletal injury. Anthropometric data (Clauser, 1969) indicate that the human skull represents approximately 7 percent of total body weight (11 pounds for a 70 kg man and 9 pounds for a 55 kg female). Relatively sedentary individuals confined to desk work or required to drive or fly for several hours per week are succeptable to postural deviations induced by lack of flexibility. In the standard desk posture, the force of gravity and weight of the head exert a downward pull of approximately 9 to 11 pounds on the musculature of the neck and upper back. Prolonged exposure to this posture can cause atrophy of the neck and back musculature, forward extension of the neck and a rounding of the shoulders and upper back. When this individual rises to an erect position, the postural changes induced by prolonged sitting tend to position the head so that the line of vision is forward and downward. In order to enhance vision, the individual contracts neck muscles that attach the back of the skull to the vertebral column. Contraction of these muscles elevates the face, enhances vision and produces a "C-shaped" curve in the region of the 3rd and 5th cervical vertebrae. With time, these muscles hypertrophy and shorten. Forward vision is maintained, the head and jaw are thrust forward, the neck is curved, cervicle (neck) mobility is reduced and the individual is prone to neck and shoulder pain. Alleviation of this problem requires the development of muscular symmetry in the muscles of the affected area. Sample rehabilitation exercises for this and other postural problems are presented in Figure 13.

Another example of postural induced problems resulting from lack of flexibility

FIGURE 13   106

NECK, SHOULDER AND BACK EXERCISES

1. Relax with knees bent and soles of feet
   together. Hold for 20 - 30 seconds.

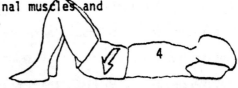

2. With back of head on the floor, turn the chin toward the
   shoulder and hold 5 - 10 seconds each side.

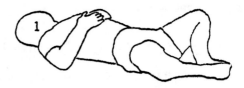

3. Pull shoulder blades together, flatten lower back
   and tighten buttocks. Hold 5 - 10 seconds, relax
   and pull head forward to stretch the back of the
   neck and upper back.

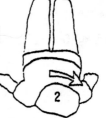

4. Tighten buttock muscles, tighten abdominal muscles and
   flatten low back. Hold 5 - 10 seconds.

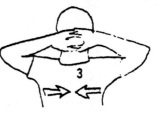

5. Extend arms overhead
   and straighten out
   legs. Stretch as far as
   possible with limbs and hold
   for 5 - 10 seconds.

FIGURE 13 contd.

107

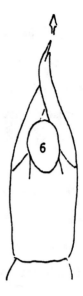

6. Stretch arms upward and backwards. Breath in as you stretch. Hold 5 - 10 seconds.

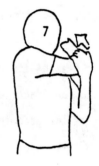

7. Gently pull elbow across the chest toward the opposite shoulder. Hold 10 - 15 seconds.

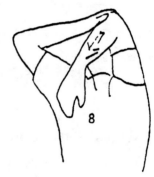

8. Gently pull elbow behind the head. Hold 10 - 15 seconds.

is low backache   Kraus and Raab (1961) estimate that 80 percent of all backache
in the U.S. is the result of muscular atrophy.   That is, 8 out of 10 cases of back -
ache are due to muscular deficiency and only 2 of 10 are the result of pathological
problems.   Industry, estimates that backache costs America one billion dollars per
year in productivity and causes 6 million Americans each day to seek medical or
therapeutic relief from pain (Keelor, 19).   Backache is the single largest drain
on employee insurance programs, accounting for approximately .25 billion dollars
per year in workmen's compensation claims.   If, as Kraus and Raab (1961) claim, most
cases of backache are attributable to muscular imbalances (Figure 14), then 3 to
5 minutes of daily strength-flexibility exercises could eliminate 80 percent of
backache , increase work output by approximately $800 billion per year, reduce
insurance claims by $20 million per year and free 4.8 million Americans from needless
aches and pains.

Lack of flexibility can contribute to back pain in at least two principle ways.
First, the common practice of using straight-leg sit-ups and leg raises to strengthen
the muscles of the abdominal area causes postural changes which enhance the possibility
of back problems. Specifically, these exercises strengthen the iliopsoas muscles
which connect the ilium (hip bone) to the femur (thigh). As this muscle becomes
stronger, it shortens and pulls the pelvis forward and downward. Since the abdominal
muscles are relatively inactive in the two aforementioned exercises, they remain too
weak to counter-act the pull of the iliopsoas which causes the pelvis to tilt
forward. This in turn causes the vertebrae in lower back to be displaced slightly
(lordosis). The articular processes of the vertebral bodies press against one another
and pain developes in the lower area of the back (Wells, 1971)

Another group of muscles associated with back pain is the hamstring group which
lie along the posterior aspect of the thigh and are responsible for movement at the
hip and knee joints. The difficulty experienced by most persons in touching the
toes from a standing or sitting position is caused by the fact that the hamstrings
are not long enough (elastic) to permit such extreme stretching. Individuals who

FIGURE 14
CAUSES OF LOW BACK PAIN*

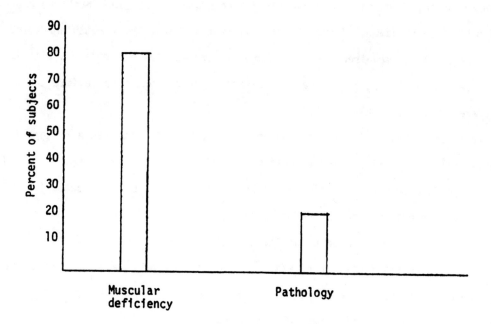

* Kraus and Raab. 1961.

spend a large amount of time sitting usually have short hamstrings. If these muscles are not stretched regularly and/or constantly held in positions that tend to shorten them, they shorten. When the individual assumes a standing position, both the knee and hip joint are extended. If the hamstrings are too short, the stretching caused by standing erect will cause direct pain in the hamstring muscles and referred pain in the low back region (Figure 15). Specific exercises to prevent or alleviate these problems are presented in Figure 16.

In addition to postural induced problems, lack of flexibility can also contribute to athletic related injuries. Individuals with limited motion in the arms and shoulders are more prone to over exertion injuries in sports such as tennis, racquetball and handball. Tight hamstrings are prone to strains (muscle pulls) and tense posterior calf muscles are related to injuries of the Achille's tendon, ankle and foot. Lack of flexibility in anterior calf muscles is associated with shin splints while tense thigh muscles (quadriceps) tend to facilitate knee problems. Specific stretching exercises for sports-type activities are presented in Chapter 7.

Increasing Flexibility. Flexibility is enhanced by stretching the musculature and connective tissue around each joint. Stretching increases range of motion, reduces muscular injuries, maintains muscular symmetry, enhances appearance, reduces muscle tension, promotes circulation and prepares the body for strenuous physical activity.

Stretching is as important for the sedentary executive, student or homemaker as it is for the most active athlete. Stretching should become an intergral part of each day. Stretching exercises can be done at any time of day: at work, in a car, standing in line, before vigorous exercise or while watching TV. Most of us are aware of the value of stretching before exercise, but have failed to recognize the importance of exercising throughout the day. In the morning, stretching increases circulation, promotes flexibility and prepares you to meet the day. Stretching at work helps release nervous tension and minimize postural deviations. Prolonged sitting or standing causes the blood to pool in the lower extremeties, increases

FIGURE 15
HAMSTRING LENGTH AND LOW BACK PAIN*

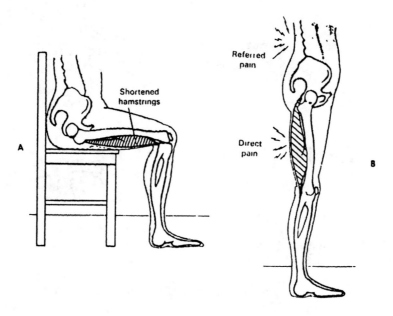

A, Position of the hamstring muscle group in relation to the bone
structure when in a sitting posture. If much of the time is spent
sitting, this muscle group may become much shorter than it should
be. B, Effect that a shortening of the hamstring muscles has on
the pelvis; when one assumes an upright standing position.
(Drawings by Eugene Sinervo; adapted from Johnson et al.)

* Hockey, 1973

FIGURE 16

LOW BACK EXERCISES

1. Pull and hold for 30 seconds.

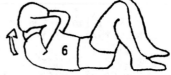

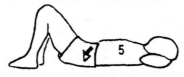

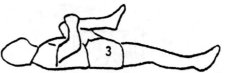

2. Relax and hold for 30 seconds.

3. Pull knee to chest and hold for 15 seconds each leg. Keep back and neck flat.

4. Pull shoulder blades together and hold for 5 - 10 seconds.

5. Tighten stomach and flatten low back on the floor. Hold 6 - 10 seconds.

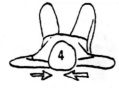

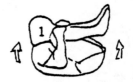

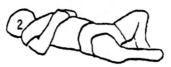

6. Curl head and shoulders 4 - 6 inches off the floor and hold for 6 - 10 seconds.

8. Stretch both arms and legs. Hold for 5 -10 seconds

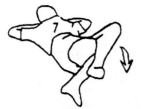

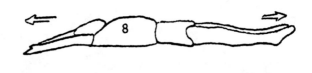

7. Cross leg over the knee and pull bottom leg toward the floor. Hold for 20 - 30 seconds.

tension and joint stiffness. Simple stretching exercises while driving or during rest breaks can reverse these changes, improve mental outlook and enhance physical comfort. Stretching at odd times during the day such as when watching TV, listening to music, reading, etc., will increase flexibility, reduce fatigue and improve mental alertness.

Most athletes would never engage in athletic competition prior to engaging in extensive warm-up/stretching exercises. Few of these athletes; however, would think to stretch during or after competition. deVries (1974) studied the EMG (electromyogram of subjects during and after exhaustive arm exercise. EMG activity (index of muscular activity) and muscle soreness increased progressively for 24 to 48 hours after cessation of exercise. Forty-eight hours after exercise the muscles were statically stretched and significant decreases in electrical activity and muscle soreness were noted. Experimental and practical experience suggests that the practice of stretching before exercise (warm-up) and after exercise (cool-down) increases circulation, improves coordination, prevents muscle injury, reduces muscle tension and facilitates recovery.

Sheehan (1978) recommends that distance runners stretch before, during and after training. Runners are encouraged to stop at 20 to 30 minute intervals to stretch the muscles of the neck, shoulders, back and legs. Training over-develops the prime movers. In running, these are the muscles along the back of the leg, thigh and low back. During exercise, these muscles fatigue and become short and inflexible. Stretching during activity will help relieve fatigue, maintain flexibility and reduce the potential for injury. With chronic exercise, the prime movers hypertrophy (grow), shorten and become tense. Daily stretching will lengthen the muscles and alleviate acute and chronic musculo-skeletal problems associated with training.

This writer recommends that 3 to 5 minutes each morning be devoted to stretching (Figure 17). Three to 5 minutes of appropriate stretching exercises should also be performed both before and after training. In addition, individuals should stretch in the middle of training runs, between sets of tennis or between games of handball,

FIGURE 17

MORNING STRETCHING EXERCISES

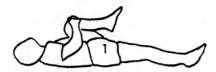

1. Pull knee to chest and hold for 15 seconds each leg. Keep back and neck flat.

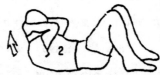

2. Curl head and shoulders 4 - 6 inches off the floor and hold for 6 -10 seconds

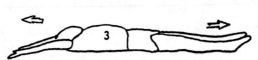

3. Stretch both arms and legs. Hold for 5 - 10 seconds.

4. Rotate each ankle clockwise and counter-clockwise through complete range of motion 10 times.

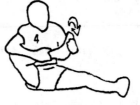

5. Pull opposite heel to buttocks with opposite hand. Hold for 20 - 30 seconds each leg.

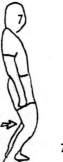

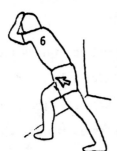

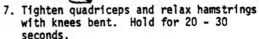

8. With knees slightly bent, relax arms and neck and bend forward at the waist. Hold for 20 - 30 seconds.

6. Keep rear heel flat. Slowly move hips forward. Hold for 20 - 30 seconds each leg.

7. Tighten quadriceps and relax hamstrings with knees bent. Hold for 20 - 30 seconds.

racquetball, etc. Individuals with limited amounts of free time might reserve the bulk of stretching (10-15 minutes) as a pre-bed time activity. Stretching before bed in front of the TV is relaxing, increases flexibility and is an economic use of time.

Stretching. Stretching exercises generally fall into one of two categories: static or dynamic (ballistic) activities. Static stretching, similar to that used in Yoga, involves holding a static position for a specified period of time. With static stretching, the specified joints are locked into a position that places the muscles and connective tissue passively at their greatest length.

The antagonist of static stretching is dynamic or ballistic stretching. Conventional calisthenic exercises usually involve jerky movements (bobbing and bouncing) in which one segment of the body is put in movement by the active contraction of a muscle group. The momentum of the moving mass is then arrested by the antagonist at the end of the range of motion. The antagonists are stretched by the dynamic movements caused by the antagonists. Since momentum is involved, the movement is called ballistic. Ballistic stretching elicits a myotatic stretch reflex to prevent the muscle from being damaged by being over-stretched (deVries, 1974). This reflex precipitates contraction of the antagonist and limits the range of motion. An example of the stretch reflex is seen when one falls asleep while setting and the head nods (neck flexes), causing the neck extensor muscles to be suddenly stretched. The stretch reflex responds (jerks) and returns the head to the erect position. The momentum generated in ballistic movements such as bobbing to touch the toes can become rather large. When this action forces the muscle to reach its maximum capacity for stretch, the stretch reflex is activated and the muscle contracts to prevent muscle damage (strain). If the momentum generated (bouncing to touch the toes) is greater than the contractile force produced by the stretch reflex, the muscle is forced to stretch beyond its limits and muscle injury can occur. Slow static stretching does not activate the stretch reflex and thus the possibility of tissue damage associated with ballistic stretching is reduced. In addition, static stretching requires less energy and is effective in both the prevention and relief of residual muscle soreness.

How to Stretch.

When stretching, you do not have to push yourself or attempt to go farther each day. You should not compare your results with those of colleagues or attempt to reach/exceed an absolute standard (Anderson, 1980). Stretching should be adjusted to fit your capabilities and needs. It should feel good when done properly and hurt when done incorrectly. The objective is to reduce muscular tension and achieve free movement, not to attain extreme flexibility. Over-achievement often leads to overstretching and injury. As previously indicated, holding a stretch as far as you can and bouncing strains the muscles and activates the stretch reflex. The end result is pain and microscopic tearing of muscle tissue. Tearing leads to the formation of scar tissue in the muscles, which causes soreness and restricts movement. The key to achieving flexibility is relaxation and regularity.

Stretching is relatively simple, but there exists both a right and wrong way to stretch. The correct method utilizes a relaxed, sustained stretch. Attention should be focused on the muscle(s) being stretched. The incorrect method emphasizes bouncing (ballistic movements) or effort to the point of pain.

According to Anderson (1980), stretching is a continuum ranging from easy to drastic stretching (Figure 18). Initial efforts should utilize an easy, sustained stretch. Participants should stretch to the point where a feeling of mild tension is observed. At this point, you should consciously attempt to relax and hold the stretch for 10-30 seconds. As the position is held, you should gradually feel the tension subside. If the tension does not subside, you should ease-off until a more comfortable degree of tension is attained. Easy stretching is designed to reduce muscular tension and prepare the tissues for the next phase, the developmental stretch.

FIGURE 18
STRETCHING CONTINUUM*

```
X ——————————————— A STRETCH ——————————————— X

X----- An Easy Stretch -------X-------The Developmental-------X-------A Drastic Stretch-----X
                                      Part of Stretching

        (hold for 20-30 seconds)     (hold for 30 seconds          (do not stretch in the
                                          or longer)                    drastic stretch)
```

* Anderson, 1980.

From the easy stretch, one gradually progresses into the developmental stretch. Stretching is extended a fraction of an inch or so until a new level of mild tension is observed. This position is held for 10-30 seconds as the tension gradually subsides. As in the easy stretch, failure to observe a reduction in tension signals the need to ease-off. This stage fine tunes the muscles and increases flexibility.

Breathing should be slow and rhythmical. Subjects should exhale as they stretch and breath slowly as the position is maintained. Under no circumstances should the breath be held during stretching. If posture inhibits natural breathing, you should ease-up, relax and try again.

CHAPTER 7

EXERCISE PRECAUTIONS AND CONTRAINDICATIONS

Medical Clearance.

Prior to getting started, there are some precautions that should be considered to ensure that training is safe, enjoyable and effective. Individuals over 35 years of age and those under 35 with one or more risk factors for coronary heart disease (smoking, obesiety, hypertension, serum lipidemia or family history) should undergo a physician monitored graded exercise stress test prior to initiating a physical fitness program (ACSM, 1975). Physical examinations and resting electro- cardiograms are often not sufficient. Studies by Cooper (1978) indicate that 1 in 10 assymptomatic adult males with normal resting electrocardiograms, have abnormal stress electrocardiograms.

The importance of coronary risk factors is illustrated in a second study by Cooper (1980). Forty-eight adult males, mean age 52.5 years, were examined for body composition, health history, exercise tolerance (CXT) and blood chemistry. These men were followed for 2 years. During this time, 15 died suddenly, 23 experienced a myocardial incident and 10 underwent by-pass surgery. Inspection of medical data revealed the following:

1) 12 had abnormal resting ECGs

2) 12 had fasting blood sugar levels greater than 110 mg%

3) 23 had cholesterol levels in excess of 250 mg%

4) 30 had a family history of heart disease

5) 16 had systolic/diastolic blood pressure readings over 140/90 mmHg

6) 32 were more than 19% fat

7) 21 smoked

8) 33 were in poor aerobic condition (less than 15 minutes on the threadmill, Balke protocol)

9) 15 had triglyceride levels in excess of 115 mg%

10) 35 had a positive stress ECG

These data indicate that heart disease has a multifocal etiology. Individuals with one or more risk factors should exercise caution before embarking on a fitness program. Exercise produces physiological stress. Individuals should be evaluated in terms of their ability to tolerate strenuous exercise on the basis of test results and an exercise prescription should be prepared that is within the safe tolerance limits of the participant. Data from Dallas (1978) indicate that individuals who receive medical clearnace, follow an exercise prescription, and observe appropriate pre-cautions significantly alter fitness with minimum risk.

Exercise prescriptions are based on individual test results and provide information related to appropriate mode of exercise as well as intensity, frequency and duration of training. Training intensity is set at an appropriate percentage of maximal heart rate. Frequency is stated as times per week and duration is expressed as minutes per day. The purpose of the exercise prescription is to ensure safe, enjoyable progress.

Clothing.

The selection of appropriate clothing is an important, but often overlooked, factor in ensuring success in a training program. The most important piece of clothing in most activities is shoes. Some podiatrists emphasize that man functions from the feet up. Defects originating in the foot can cause problems in other areas such as the knee, hip, and back, sufficient to impede or stop training.

Different types of shoes are designed for specific purposes. Sneakers, made for games and sports, are not only ineffective, but are often the principle cause of prin and injury when used for jogging. Likewise, jogging shoes which are not designed for competitive sports are often the cause of ankle and knee injuries in basketball and racuqet sport participants.

When choosing a sport shoe, examine all models (figures estimate that 45 percent of all shoes currently manufactured in the world are athletic in design) and limit choeces to those designed specifically for your needs. That is, tennis players should examine tennis shoes, joggers should evaluate running shoes, etc. Irresnective of design, the primary requirements of all shoes should be fit and support. Shoes should be fit, if possible, at approximately the same time of day that they will be used. Since the feet tend to swell with time, it would be foolish to fit a pair of shoes at 8:00 AM for use at 5:00 PM. When fitting shoes, wear athletic socks identical to those that will be worn in training. Lace both shoes and walk/jog around the store. Try to subject the shoes to movements similar to those that will be required of the sport or activity for which they are being purchased. Quality control in some models is less than ideal and variability exists among brands with respect to length and width. Disregard sizes and fit the shoes to your feet.

Because of the proliferation of runners and running shoes, guidelines have been developed for the selection of running shoes (1978). First, purchase shoes from a store that caters to runners and has one or more experienced runners on staff. Next, limit selections to well-known brands that have been subjected to independent investigations. Runner's World magazine periodically evaluates running shoes and rates them 1 to 5-star. In general, shoes rated 4 or 5 star are the best buys. A list of 4 and 5 star shoes for 1979 is presented in Table 27. Be prepared to spend at least $25 for a pair of good running shoes. A number of shoes are more expensive, but most runners are satisfied with medium priced shoes.

Good running form dictates that the foot contact the ground either heel first or flat footed. Because of this strike pattern, the outer border of the heel of most running shoes wears rather quickly. Smart runners pruchase a tube of shoe-goo or shoe patch (approximately $3-4.00) with each pair of shoes. Weekly application of these substances will minimize heel wear and extend the life of the shoes by several hundred miles. A tube of shoe-goo will last most runners approximately 12 months and delay the need to purchase new shoes.

Running shoes, like all other shoes, are built on a mold or last. The sole is the superstructure upon which the shoe is built. The outer sole is that protion that makes contact with the ground and the part that wears out. The midsole is that

TABLE 27

RATINGS FOR RUNNING SHOES*

Rating (stars)	Men's Shoes	Women's Shoes
5	Saucony Hornet	Brooks Lady Vantage
5	Nike LDV	Brooks Lady Vantage Supreme
5	New Balance 320	Tiger Tigress
5	New Balance Trail 355	New Balance W 320
5	Saucony Trainer 1980	
5	Converse WC Trainer II	
5	Brooks Vantage	
5	Brooks Vantage Supreme	
4	Converse Arizona	Saucony Dove - 2
4	Osaga Caliente	Osaga Feather
4	Brooks Delta	Adidas Lady Orion
4	Adidas Dragon	Etonic Lady Street Fighter
4	Adidas TRX Competition	Nike Lady Waffle Trainer
4	Etonic KM 501	Tred 2 Lady Zephyr
4	Adidas Orion	Saucony Ms Gripper
4	Nike Roadrunner I	Nike Senorita Cortez I
4	Etonic Street Fighter	Converse Women's WC Trainer II

* Runner's World (1979).

and is the part that, if made of cheap or bad material, can compress after several weeks and negate its beneficial characteristics. Compression of the midsole is common among discount brand running shoes. The midsole should be constructed of a flexible material that will absorb shock and make the shoe flexible.

The insole, the portion that actually comes in contact with the foot, is usually made of Spenco, rubber or leather. Spenco is the preferred material because of its shock absorption characteristics. In addition to shock absorption, insoles are designed to eliminate blisters caused by rubbing and sliding. Cloth insoles should be avoided as they tend to irritate and absorb perspiration like a sponge Arch supports are built into most shoes and should be removed by individuals wearing orthodics.

Soles come in various thicknesses, layers and patterns. Design patterns range from smooth to waffels. While some designers claim that their sole patterns are superior for shock absorption, stability, wear, etc., scientific study (Higdon, 1978) indicates that most patterns vary only with respect to traction. Stud-type soles offer better traction on soft surfaces, but tend to slide on wet asphalt. Individuals who run on grass might be better satisfied with stud-type shoes. Some street runners prefer ripple or herring-bone (transverse) patterns. Most patterns are effective for street wear. Problems usually occur only when conditions are wet and soles are extremely worn. Runners are advised to replace shoes when sole wear becomes extreme. Excessive sole wear reduces traction, decreases shock absorption capability and places the foot in a posture that is conducive to musculoskeletal injury.

Soles are designed to absorb shock, maintain stability and provide traction. Choose soles that are light, flexible, have a good midsole, provide some form of transverse or stud design and have a high predicted life expectancy. Each of these characteristics is evaluated in the annual October Runner's World shoe survey.

The foxing is the material portion of the shoe that gives medial and lateral support. It is usually made of suede and runs around the heel and toe area. The toe cap (toe box), the foxing that covers the toe area, is designed to prevent scuffing and rubbing of the toes against the shoe. The heel counter, rear foxing, stabilizes the heel by minimizing the pronatory forces that are transmitted to the heel at contact. The protrusion above the heel is the pull tab used to help pull on the shoe.

The toe box is essential for long distance running. Shoes should be fitted from heel to toe and selected so that at least .25 inch of extra length is available between the end of the shoe and the longest toe. This extra room minimizes the chances of blisters, allows the foot to swell (feet will swell to a size and one-half over normal) and enables the foot to shift forward in the shoe when running downhill.

The heel counter is an extremely important aspect in shoe design. It should be constructed of rigid material and extend as far as possible to minimize the pronation and supination forces at the heel. A soft heel counter leads to rotational injuries of the lower leg, knee and hip. A rigid heel counter prevents the foot from twisting or turning in the heel area on contact. The material under the heel should be slightly elevated and able to withstand relatively high impact forces. Slight elevation of the heel minimizes Achille's tendon pain and injury. The heel counter should fit snugly around the heel.

The upper is the material that covers the top of the foot and gives the shoe its color and aesthetic appeal. Uppers are usually made of nylon for lightness, nylon mesh for coolness and airflow or leather for bad weather. Nylon is lighter and less abrasive than leather and does not take on the shape of the foot. Leather molds to the shape of the foot and runners with pronated ankles (turn in) are habitually subjected to excess shoe force. Leather also retains more moisture than nylon which drys and leaves potentially abrasive salt deposits.

In addition to shoes, other pieces of clothing are essential for effective and comfortable training. Individuals should make a habit of wearing cotton socks or low cut tennis-style cotton socks when training. Aside from problems related to hygiene and fungus, socks minimize abrasion between the feet and shoes. Cotton absorbs perspiration, adds cushioning and minimizes the wear on the shoes caused by excessive exposure to salt and moisture. Nylon socks retain heat and moisture and can contribute to blisters. Wool socks tend to be thicker, heavier and hotter than cotton.

During mild to hot weather, participants should wear shorts and a T-shirt. Cotton or cotton-blend shorts are good, but tend to get heavy with perspiration and the thick in-seam can cause abrasions on the inner side of the thighs. A good alternative is the quick drying, light weight, running shorts made of 100 percent stretch nylon tricot. These shorts are soft, resist binding, rubbing and chafing. They come in a variety of colors. Many contain a built-in brief and some are uni-sex.

Individuals with heavy thighs, especially those who train in cotton shorts, should purchase a tube of Vaseline petroleum jelly and Destine anti-diaper rash. A liberal application of vaseline to the thighs will minimize rubbing and chafing. Should chafing occur, the application of Destine between runs is extremely effective in promoting healing. Individuals prone to chafing and those too chafed to workout are often delighted to find that they can prevent chafing, eliminate pain and return to training by simply wearing panty hose under their workout clothing. Panty hose are sometimes hot, but they provide free, painless movement.

Light-weight cotton or cotton-blend T-shirts are recommended for training. Cotton absorbs perspiration, facilitates cooling and minimizes abrasions. Individuals working in the sun should wear light colored shirts that reflect the sun rays.

Women are sometimes confused about the necessity for bras. The amount of support needed from a bra depends upon body build (Ullyot, 1976). Women with small chests may be perfectly comfortable training without a bra. Large breasted women usually need the support of a sturdy bra. Light-weight running-athletic bras are commerically available.

Clothing and Environment.

Participants, especially runners, should consider the weather when dressing. On cold days, clothing should be applied in layers of T-shirts and sweatshirts and a light jacket should be worn. The outer layers of clothing should contain snaps, zippers, etc, down the front that allow you to regulate heat build-up. As body heat increases, remove one layer at a time and tie the extra clothing around your waist. Sweat pants, long underwear, tights or panty hose should be worn on the legs. Knit hats or ski caps are effective in keeping the head and ears warm. Wool gloves, mittens and sweat socks are useful for keeping the hands warm.

Some individuals, especially runners, express a fear having their lungs freeze in very cold weather. No evidence exists to suggest that cold can cause injury to the larynx, bronchi or lungs. Air inspired at 40° below zero (^oF), is 50-60° F by the time it reaches the mouth. The extreme dryness of cold air may lead to temporary cracking and bleeding of the respiratory passages. Individuals required to train in cold weather might consult the following guide in Table 28 as an aid to select proper clothing.

Monitor the temperture, sun rays, humidity and wind velocity. On calm, sunny days, shorts and a T-shirt are usually satisfactory if the temperature is above 50 degrees. After 5-6 minutes, body temperature increases and sweat suits often become too hot. Rubberized clothing is an absolute contraindication irrespective of the weather. Body heat can build-up to dangerous levels in individuals who train in rubber suits. Cotton sweats should not be worn as outer garments in the rain. They absorb water, become heavy and sag. Water proof wind breakers and rain jackets are recommended for rainy weather. Hats and hoods keep the rain off the head, but create an environment in which body heat causes the head to become wet with perspiration. After the workout, get warm and dry as soon as possible. A hot bath or shower is the perfect ending to a rainy day workout.

The dangers of heat can not be over emphasized. Body temperature increases

TABLE 28
GUIDELINES FOR RUNNING IN COLD WEATHER*

WIND-CHILL READINGS								
Temperature (Farenheit)								
Calm	40	35	30	25	20	15	10	5
Equivalent Chill Temperature								
5	35	30	25	20	15	10	5	0
10	30	20	15	10	5	0	-10	-15
15	25	15	10	0	-5	-10	-20	-25
20	20	10	5	0	-10	-15	-25	-30
25	15	10	0	-5	-15	-20	-30	-35
30	10	5	0	-10	-20	-25	-30	-40
35	10	5	-5	-10	-20	-25	-35	-40
40	10	0	-5	-15	-20	-30	-35	-45

WIND (M.P.H.) is the left-hand vertical axis for the wind values above.

Little Danger   Increasing Danger

(Farenheit)								
0	-5	-10	-15	-20	-25	-30	-35	-40
Equivalent Chill Temperature								
-5	-10	-15	-20	-25	-30	-35	-40	-45
-20	-25	-35	-40	-45	-50	-60	-65	-70
-30	-40	-45	-50	-60	-65	-70	-80	-85
-35	-45	-50	-60	-65	-75	-80	-85	-95
-45	-50	-60	-65	-75	-80	-90	-95	-105
-50	-55	-65	-70	-80	-85	-95	-100	-105
-50	-60	-65	-75	-80	-90	-100	-105	-115
-55	-60	-70	-75	-85	-95	-100	-110	-115

Increasing Danger
(Flesh may freeze within one minute)

Great Danger
(Flesh may freeze within 30 seconds)

* Sheehan. 1978.

with exercise and this heat must be eliminated if thermal balance and physical health are to be maintained. Heat can kill, especially when the humidity is high. The data in Figure 19 was devised for individuals who must train in hot, humid weather. Individuals who exercise at high temperatures and humidity levels are extremely prone to heat illness. It is important to note that similar heat problems can occur when the weather is cool and the humidity is high. Overexertion at moderate temperatures and high humidity can be as dangerous as overexertion at higher temperatures. Guidelines for exercise in the heat are presented in Table 29.

The body's chief avenues of heat loss are conduction, convection, radiation and evaporation. Cooling by conduction, touching an object cooler than you are, is impossible during the summer in the South. Convection, the passing of cool air across the body, is also limited in the summer. If the air is cooler than the body (as in a fan), temperature will decrease. However, if the air temperature is higher than body temperature, the body will become hotter. Radiation is the absorption of heat rays. On clear or partly cloudy days, the sun's rays can significantly elevate body temperature. The most effective method of cooling the body is evapora-tion, the process of changing moisture (sweat) to a gas and thereby releasing body heat. On humid days, the air is moist and evaporation is severely reduced. During summer months in the South all avenues of cooling; conduction, convection, radiation and evaporation, can be severely restricted.

During exercise, the body acts as a machine and converts chemical energy into mechanical energy in the muscles. The human body is an extremely inefficient machine and releases approximately 70 percent of the total energy generated as heat. In order to maintain thermal balance, this heat must be dissipated via or more of the aforementioned methods. Failure to completely dissipate all of the heat generated, causes body temperature to rise to dangerous levels and precipitates heat illness and/or death.

As exercise begins, heart rate rises to increase the flow of blood to the working

FIGURE 19

HEAT SAFETY INDEX*

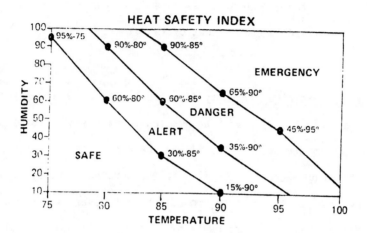

* Sheehan. 1978.

muscles. Flow to non-essential muscles is reduced and shunted to the working muscles and to the skin. As the blood flows toward the skin, the vessels near the surface dilate and skin becomes flush. At the skin's surface, circulating air currents convect the heat away, heat waves are radiated to cooler objects in the environment and/or surface heat is used to evaporate perspiration lying on the skin. The efficiency of each of these mechanisms is dependent upon a number of factors, most of which can be modified to some extent by the participant. These factors include:

Exercise Intensity. As exercise intensity increases, heart rate rises and the body either; (1) pumps more blood to the working muscles to maintain performance or (2) diverts blood flow to the skin to facilitate the dissipation of body heat. Most of the time, the body increases the flow to the working muscles. This process enables us to increase or sustain energy production, but severely restricts our ability to loose heat. With sustained exercise, effective thermoregulation becomes dependent upon environmental conditions. If environmental conditions are unfavorable, the participant must reduce or cease activity. Failure to decrease effort will cause heat to accumulate until body temperature reaches the critical level at which heat illness occurs.

Temperature, Wind Speed and Humidity. Temperature and wind speed influence the amount of heat dissipated by convection. High wind speeds cause a larger volume of air to cross the body and increases the potential for heat loss. Heat loss will occur if the air temperature is less than that of the skin. Movement produces wind speed which can effectively aid-heat loss. In general, the higher the body speed, the greater the potential for heat loss. Since cyclists travel at faster speeds than runners, they usually have fewer problems with heat illness.

As the air becomes more humid, the medium for evaporation decreases and the body looses its ability to evaporate perspiration. Perspiration continues to drop from the body, fluid loss increases and dehydration begins. If activity is not ceased and fluid replaced, a critical physiological situation will insue; (1) water will be diffused from the blood plasma to maintain cellular equilibrium, (2) loss of water will reduce the circulating blood volume, (3) heart rate will increase to distribute the reduced blood volume, (4) loss of water will diminish the capacity of the blood to dilute the electrolyte concentration in the blood, (5) as water losses become excessive, the sweating mechanism will be turned off to maintain blood volume, bocy temperature will rise to dangerous levels (104-105°F) and heat shock will occur, and (6) the high concentration of electrolytes in the blood will interfer with the normal rhythm of the heart and can precipitate ventricular fibrillation, heart failure and death.

The relationship between intensity of exercise and environmental conditions is depicted in Figure 20. Twenty adult male runners were monitored for physiological responses (heart rate, oxygen uptake, ventilation rate, core temperature, skin temperature and sweat loss) as they ran at different percentages of maximum capacity under 3 environmental conditions. Each subject ran for 30 minutes on a motor-driven treadmill located in an environmental chamber. Treadmill speeds were selected to represent approximately 75 and 85 percent of aerobic capacity. Environmental conditions were selected to represent different combinations of wet bulb (humidity), dry bulb (ambient temperature) and black bulb (radiant load) temperatures. Wet bulb-globe indices (WBGT) of 70, 80 and 90°F were used as environmental loads. WBGT indicies were calculated according to procedures established by the military (Fox, 1979), where WBGT = (.7 X WB + .1 X DB + .2 X BB). Ambient temperature and relative humidity were produced by the environmental chamber. Radiant load was established through the use of heat lamps. Wind speed was set at running speed. Wind speed and circulation were simulated through the use of fans.

As expected, the results indicated that all physiological responses increases with intensity of effort and thermal load. In addition, thermal stress was influenced

FIGURE 20

HEAT, ACTIVITY AND CORE TEMPERATURE

75% - 70° F
75% - 80° F
75% - 90° F
85% - 70° F
85% - 80° F
85% - 90° F

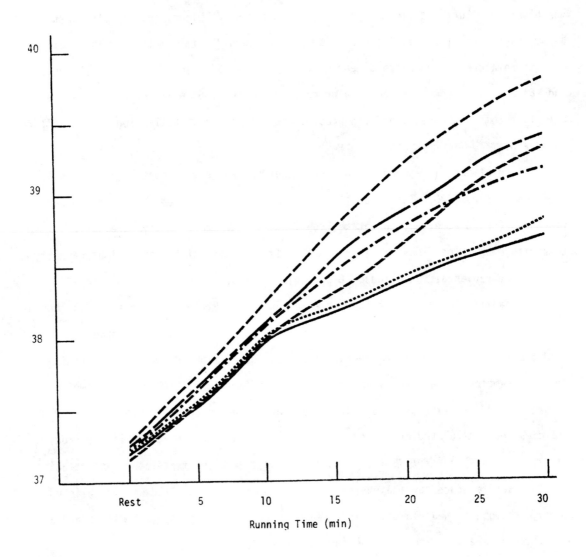

Running Time (min)

more by environmental condition than by work intensity. Comparison of the curve depicting 75 percent effort at 90°F WBGT with that for 85 percent effort at 70°F WBGT indicates that mild work at extreme environments was more stressful than moderate work at mild environments. Thus, individuals exercising in extreme environments must reduce the intensity of effort and utilize frequent rest and fluid breaks.

Research indicates that athletes can loose 1-2 liters of sweat every hour. Heavier athletes tend to loose more. If fluid is not replaced, dehydration occurs. Wyndham and Strydom (1969) has shown that core temperature and the risk of heat illness increase as fluid loss approaches 3 percent of total body weight. For this reason, individuals are encouraged to drink liberal quanities of fluid before, during and after activity. Because of the increasing potential for heat illness among runners, the ACSM has published the following "Guidelines For Exercising (running) in the Heat."

Individuals exercising in hot weather are instructed to consume large quanities of fluids. Research by Costill (1978) indicates that consumption of fluids before, during and after exercise will minimize the degree of dehydration that normally results from prolonged sweating and reduce circulatory stress. The data in Figure 21 indicates that drinking water during 2 hours of cycling in the heat has a dramatic effect on the volume of plasma when compared to the same condition performed without fluids. The end result is the availability of more blood for transportation of essential nutrients to the working muscles and to transfer heat to the preiphery of the body.

Water does not go directly from the stomach to the blood. It must first pass into the intestine where absorption can occur rather rapidly. The major limitations to fluid replacement appears to be how fast the solution leaves the stomach (rate of gastric emptying). Costill (1978) has determined that factors such as the volume, temperature and sugar content of a drink can affect the rate of gastric emptying.

Research indicates that large volumes (up to 600 ml) leave the stomach more rapidly than small ones, but subjects usually complain that large volumes are uncomfortable, distend the stomach and interfer with respiratory movements. A

TABLE 29

GUIDELINES FOR EXERCISE IN THE HEAT*

"Distance races (16 kilometers, or 10 miles) should not be conducted when the wet bulb globe termperature exceeds 82.4°F. (28.0°C).

"During periods of the year when the daylight dry bulb temperature often exceeds 80°F. (27°C.), distance races should be conducted before 9 AM or after 4 PM.

"It is the responsibility of the race sponsors to provide fluids which contain small amounts of sugar (less than 2.5 grams of glucose per 100 ml of water) and electrolytes (less than 10 milliequivalents or 230 mg of sodium and 5 milliequivalents or 195 mg of potassium per liter of solution).

"Runners should be encouraged to frequently ingest fluids during competition and to consume 400 to 500 ml (13 to 17 ounces) of fluid 10 to 15 minutes before competition.

"Rules prohibiting the administration of fluids during the first 6.2 miles (10 kilometers) of a marathon race should be amended to permit fluid ingestion at frequent intervals along the race course. In light of the high sweat rates and body temperatures during distance running in the heat, race sponsors should provide 'water stations' at 2- to 2½ mile (3- to 4-km) intervals for all races of 10 miles (16 km) or more.

"Runners should be instructed in how to recognize the early warning symptoms that precede heat injury. Recognition of symptoms, cessation of running, and proper treatment can prevent heat injury. Early warning symptoms include the following: piloerection (the hair stands on end) on chest and arms; chilling; throbbing pressure in the head; unsteadiness; nausea; and dry skin.

"Race sponsors should make prior arrangements with medical personnel for the care of

TABLE 29

GUIDELINES FOR EXERCISE IN THE HEAT*

"cases of heat injury. Responsible and informed personnel should supervise each 'feeding station. Organizational personnel should reserve the right to stop runners who exhibit clear signs of heat stroke or heat exhaustion."

*ACSM (1978)

FIGURE 21
EFFECTS OF DEHYDRATION ON HEART RATE
AND RECTAL TEMPERATURE DURING TWO
HOURS OF CYCLING*

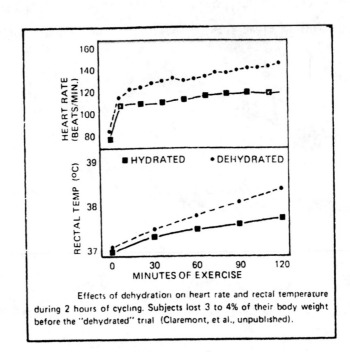

Effects of dehydration on heart rate and rectal temperature during 2 hours of cycling. Subjects lost 3 to 4% of their body weight before the "dehydrated" trial (Claremont, et al., unpublished).

*Higdon (1978)

wiser choice is to drink 150-250 ml (5-8.5 ozs.) at 10-15 minute intervals. Cold fluids leave the stomach more rapidly and are more effective than warm fluids for cooling the body. Likewise, the type of fluid injested also affects the speed at which fluid is absorbed from the stomach. Water appears to be one of the fastest substances to leave the stomach. Fluids containing sugar are the slowest to leave the stomach. Research indicates that sugar retards gastric emptying. The rate at which fluids leave the stomach is inversely related to the quanity of sugar in the drink (Figure 22). Costill (1978) has subjects drink either 400 ml (13.5 oz) of water or 400 ml of Coca-Cola containing 40 grams of sugar (sucrose). Within 15 minutes, approximately 60-70 percent of the water had left the stomach as compared to only 5 percent of the soft drink. Similar comparisons of commerical aid drinks revealed that Gatorade and other drinks high in sugar left the stomach less rapidly than did water, Break Time, ERG or Body Punch. Drinks containing high quanities of sugar are slow to leave the stomach and thus deliver relatively small quanities of water to the system. Ideally, the sugar content of replacement drinks should not exceed 2-2.5 grams per 100 milliliters of water. This does not imply that you should not drink Gatorade during activity, only that you should not drink it full strength. Mixing Gatorade with an equal volume of water dilutes the drink and reduces the sugar content per volume to acceptable levels.

While commericial drink manufacturers emphasize the importance of replacing electrolytes during activity, recent research questions the need for such practices. Costill (1978) contends that the body has the ability to minimize electrolyte losses during strenuous exercise and dehydration. He suggests that electrolyte loss during activity is minimal and can be adequately replaced post-exercise through sound dietary practices.

Most authorities condemn the use of salt tablets before or after exercise. Rather, they recommend the addition of salt through normal dietary means. Salt tablets, unless taken with large amounts of fluids (approximately 1 pint of water per 7-grain tablet), can slow the absorption process and may aggravate heat stress

FIGURE 22

EFFECT OF GLUCOSE CONCENTRATION IN A
SOLUTION ON THE RATE OF GASTRIC EMPTYING*

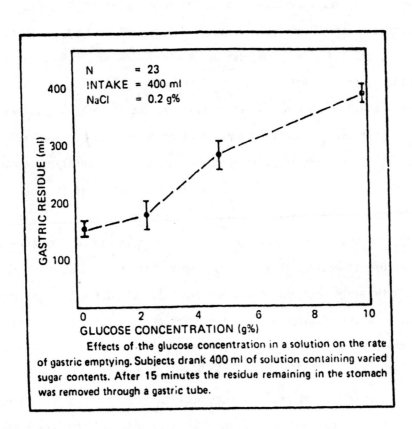

Effects of the glucose concentration in a solution on the rate of gastric emptying. Subjects drank 400 ml of solution containing varied sugar contents. After 15 minutes the residue remaining in the stomach was removed through a gastric tube.

* Higdon (1978)

problems. Inspection of Table 30 indicates that replacement of salt is contra-
indicated until fluid loss reaches approximately 8 pounds or pints.

The "Guidelines For The Drinking Athlete" (Table 31) were established by Costill
(1978) and should be observed by all individuals performing exercise in the heat:
Individuals accustomed to drinking electrolyte replacement drinks might find the
following receipt to be an effective, low cost substitute for the more expensive
commerical drinks (Sheehan, 1978):

1 gallon water

1 tablespoon iodized salt

3 tablespoons sugar

1 package koolaide

Air Pollution and Altitude. A serious environmental concern among residents or
urban areas is air pollution. Typical pollutants in most cities include particulate
matter, ozone and carbon monoxide. Most newpapers publish daily indices of pollutant
levels. Individuals with respiratory problems should refer to these periodically.
According to Sheehan (1978), the body will tell you when pollution levels are too
high to exercise. The development of symptoms such as eye and respiratory irritation and/or disruption of normal vision are signs that the air quality is too poor to
support safe training.

Research in California and Japan indicate that pollution, especially ozone and
petrochemical smog will decrease physical performance and exercise tolerance.
Fortunately, these distrubances are temporary in healthy individuals. Subjects
with chronic respiratory disorders; however, should avoid exercise when air quality
decreases.

Altitude is another factor that can affect aerobic performance, especially at
levels in excess of 7000 feet. As altitude increases, the heart and lungs must
work harder to compensate for the reduced pressure of oxygen. Maximum oxygen uptake is reduced by 5-25 percent during brief exposure to altitudes of 7500 feet.

TABLE 30

A GUIDE FOR SALT REPLACEMENT*

APPROXIMATE SALT LOSS				SUPPLEMENTAL REPLACEMENT	
Water Loss, Pounds or Pints	Grams	Grains	Water (Pints)	No. or 7-Grain Salt Tablets* to be taken per pint of water (Replaced)	
2	1.5	23	2	Diet adequate	
4	3.0	46	4	Diet adequate	
6	4.5	69	6	Diet adequate	
				NONACCLIMATIZED	ACCLIMATIZED
8	6.0	92	8	2	1
10	7.5	115	10	4	3
12	9.0	138	12	6	5

*Salt tablets usually come in 7- and 10-grain sizes (15.4 grains equal 1 gm).

*Mathews and Fox, (1971)

* Mathews and Fox, (1971).

TABLE 31
GUIDELINES FOR THE DRINKING ATHLETE*

During hot-weather competition and training the athlete should use the following guidelines:

1. The drink should be: (a) hypotonic (few solid particles per unit of water); (b) low in sugar concentration (less than 2.5 grams per 100 milliliters of water); (c) cold (roughly 45-55 degrees F or 8-13 degrees C); (d) consumed in volumes ranging from 100-400 milliliters (3-10 ounces); (e) palatable.

2. Drink 400-600 milliliters (13.5-20 ounces) of water or the above drink 10-15 minutes before the start of competition.

3. During the competition, 100-200 milliliters (3-6.5 ounces) of the above drink should be taken at 10-15 minute intervals throughout the activity.

4. Following the competition, eating a good meal and an effort to drink more fluids can adequately replace the electrolytes lost in sweat.

5. The athlete should keep a record of his or her early-morning body weight (taken immediately after rising, after urination and before breakfast) to detect symptoms of a condition of chronic dehydration. (If your weight is too low, you may be losing more water than you can afford to.)

6. Drinks are of significant value in races lasting more that 50 or 60 minutes. So if you like to run distance events longer than 15 kilometers, you better learn how to drink.

*Higdon (1978)

Pulmonary ventilation (rate and volume) and heart rate are significantly increased during work at altitude and dehydration becomes a problem due to the dryness of air. The end result is that maximal work capacity is reduced (Figure 23). Likewise, the physical effort required to sustain a given aerobic workload is significantly higher than that observed at sea level. These changes are temporary and the body compensates by increasing the hemoglobin and total blood volume with acclimatization.

All individuals, especially those with cardiac problems are encouraged to reduce the intensity and duration of training bouts upon exposure to altitude. Some authorities recommend a minimum of 2 days of acclimatization per 3000 feet of elevation. Exercise at elevation can be safe and productive if participants recognize the limitations and adjust their effort accordingly.

Acute Health Problems. During the year, the average individual may experience several acute health problems and become confused as to whether or not to train. Most acute problems tend to be respiratory in nature and interfere with the free flow of air. A common problem, especially during the winter months, is sore throat. Medical authorities suggest that sore throat, a condition due to persistent sinus infection or allergy, may be aggravated by severe exercise. Extreme levels of exercise lowers the body's ability to handle allergies and reduces its defense against infection. Participants are encouraged to see a physician before exercising with a sore throat.

Colds and Flu. Some physicians do not encourage their patients to cease exercise when afflicted with a simple head cold. Exercise often helps clear the nose and sinuses and makes the participant feel better after exercise. If you choose to workout with a cold, be careful to keep warm and avoid overexertion (fatigue). Avoiding overexertion implys that you cut back on the intensity and total work output. Runners are encouraged to reduce their daily mileage by approximately 50 percent until symptoms are relieved.

Fever. The presence of fever indicates that problems are more serious and is an

FIGURE 23

143

ALTITUDE AND AEROBIC CAPACITY

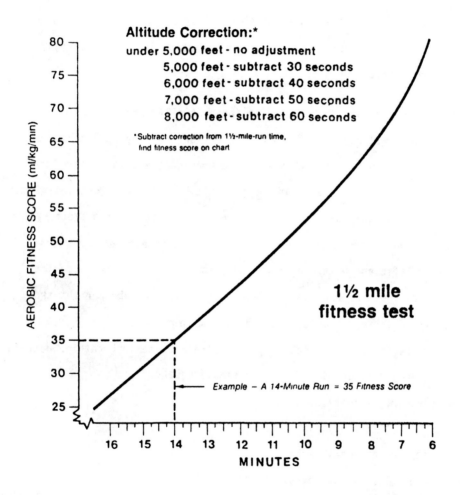

Altitude Correction:*

under 5,000 feet - no adjustment

5,000 feet - subtract 30 seconds

6,000 feet - subtract 40 seconds

7,000 feet - subtract 50 seconds

8,000 feet - subtract 60 seconds

*Subtract correction from 1½-mile-run time, find fitness score on chart

1½ mile fitness test

Example – A 14-Minute Run = 35 Fitness Score

AEROBIC FITNESS SCORE (ml/kg/min)

MINUTES

contraindication to exercise. With fever, the body is in a very weakened state, viruses may be circulating in the blood and additional stresses on the system should be avoided.

Runny Nose. Most individuals who exercise experience a runny nose   sometime during their training. Nasal secretions are beneficial for clearing sinuses and nasal pas- sages. These secretions may be the result of physical stress or irritaiton produced by increased nasal flow. Unless signs of fever or infection are present, nasal secretions should not limit exercise.

Stitches. A stitch is a rather sharp abdominal pain usually located just under the ribs on the right side. It usually occurs with exertion (running) and ceases or decreases with rest or reduction in activity. The precise cause is unknown, but is thought to be a spasm of the diaphragm due to faulty breathing. Most individuals tend to breath by raising the chest and contracting the stomach. This procedure is innefficient and common in beginning runners who have not developed an effective breathing pattern. Efficient breathing is relaxed and centered in the abdominal area. As you inhale, the diaphragm should descend and push the abdomen outward. When you exhale, the diaphragm should rise and the abdomen flatten.

Beginning runners can avoid stitches by utilizing a rhythmic breathing pattern. Breathing should be coordinated with following step frequency:

(1) First step (right foot), inhale

(2) Second step (left foot), inhale again

(3) Third step (right foot), exhale

(4) Fourth step (left foot), exhale again.

By coordinating breathing with foot strike, the runner can ensure a rhythmic, efficient rate. The process of using 2 successive inhalations and exhalations enables the runner to more completely fill and empty the lungs. Runners who sense the coming of a stitch should try to concentrate on rhythmic breathing. A good technique is to forceably make noise with each breath. Efficient runners often sound like a

train; woo-woo/choo-choo. Not all **stitches are attributable to faulty breathing.**
Some cases are related to irritation of the diaphragm caused by injesting food or
drinking too soon before exercise.

Varicose Veins. Varicose veins are due to high hydrostatic pressure in the super-
ficial (saphenous) veins of the legs. Over time, this pressure overcomes the natural
elasticity of the walls of the veins and causes the veins to bulge and distend.
Since the vein structure can not be strengthened, the key is prevention. In order
to prevent varicose veins, the hydrostatic pressure in the veins must be reduced.
This is best achieved by sitting with the feet elevated. Other approaches include
the wearing of support hose, avoidance of prolonged standing, constricting garters
and knee socks. To date, there exists no cause-effect relationship between varicose
veins and exercise (running). However, since varicose veins tend to run in families,
individuals with symptomatic parents might be wise to use exercise and avoid
situations that elevate hydrostatic pressure.

Hemorrhoids. Hemorrhoids are varicose veins of the rectum and anus and are not caused
by severe exercise. They can occur in all individuals, active and sedentary, who
have infrequent bowel movement and are constipated as a result of low intake of
fluid and dietary-fiber. While hemorrhoids can be extremely painful, there exists
no evidence that exercise can cause or cure them. The best approach is prevention.
Prevention is often achieved by consuming diets high in fiber content. Some authorities
suggest that injestion of 1 tablespoon of bran (10-15 gms) and at least 7 ounces (200
gms) of fresh fruit and vegetables will soften the stool, eliminate constipation and
prevent the development of hemorrhoids.

Menstrual problems. Most physicians permit women to exercise during the menstrual
cycle provided cramps are not too severe. While some authorities report that walking
and jogging are effective in alleviating cramps, no data exist to suggest that activity
will increase the severity of cramps or prolong bleeding. A few studies have

indicated that women who run 50 to 100 miles per week often experience a reduction or cessation of menstrual flow. Exercise physiologists speculate that this phenome non is related to the percent body fat that a woman has (Drinkwater, 1977). When the fat level is reduced below an undefined level menstruation ceases. When activity is curtailed and/or fat level increased, normal flow returns.

The most common female complaint is dysmenorrhea, painful periods. Lower abdominal pains, cramps, backache and sometimes headache, leg pain, breast fullness or tenderness and nausea generally characterize this problem. The amount of pain experienced is hard to quantify because of varying subjective factors and differences in pain tolerance among women. Gynecologists estimate that 70-80 percent of the cases of painful menstruation can be attributed to faulty living habits, e.g.,.lack of exercise, poor posture, fatigue, irritability and tension from daily activities. Studies at the various U.S. service academies indicate that dysmenorrhea is less common among healthy female athletes and physical education students than among those who are physically inactive. Likewise, women who engaged in strenuous physical activity during a two year period reported greatly reduced dysmenorrhea compared to that experienced prior to entrance into the academies.

Pregnancy. Scientific study of the effects of training during pregnancy is limited (Ullyot, 1976). Most physicians tell their patients to, "Do what you're accustomed to, as long as it feels comfortable." Women accustomed to daily jogging are usually permitted to continue. If they become fatigued, they are advised to reduce their mileage and/or walk.
Ullyot (1976) recommends that her patients use the "talk test" while running. She contends that both mother and baby will receive adequate oxygen provided the mother does not over-exert herself. Exercise increases circulation and maintains muscular tone. Most obstetricians believe that child birth is easier and post-partum recovery is faster in athletic women.

Some women fear that exercise will induce miscarriage or jar the fetus. Ullyot

(1976) says that these fears are unfounded. Early miscarriage is caused by the death of a defective ovum or fetus. The fetus is suspended in amniotic fluid which protects the fetus and cushions it against bumps and jars.

Diet Before Activity. Performance during workouts can be impaired if the participant has just eaten. Generally, there is a feeling of discomfort when one attempts heavy exertion on a full stomach. Most authorities suggest that training be avoided for at least 2-3 hours after eating. Fats and meat are slow to digest, consequently, they should not be eaten less than 3 to 4 hours before training. Recent survey of runners by Higdon (1978) indicates that most runners prefer to wait at least 2 hours after the last meal before training.

Smoking. Most Americans are aware that smoking contributes to heart disease and lung cancer. Smoking can reduce the length and quality of life. Scientific study indicates that smoking can interfere with normal breathing both at rest and during exercise. Nadel and Conroe (1961) have demonstrated that as few as 15 puffs of cigarette smoke in 5 minutes can reduce airway conductance by 31 percent in normal subjects. These changes occurred as early as one minute after smoking begins and last from 10 to 80 minutes.

The nicotine in cigarettes causes an increase in heart rate and elevation of blood pressure. Therefore, smoking increases the work of the heart and the demands of the heart muscle for oxygen. The carbon monoxide in smoke combines with hemoglobin approximately 300 times more readily than oxygen and reduces its capacity to carry oxygen. Smokers are handicapped when they perform physical activity because (1) they inhale less air per breath than non-smokers; and (2) the oxygen carrying capacity of their blood is less than that of non-smokers. Therefore, smokers are frequently short of breath and have less aerobic capacity than non-smokers. Fortunately, these limitations appear to be reversable. Data suggest that smokers who become physically fit, usually quit or significantly reduce cigarette dependence, enhance breathing efficiency and improve cardiorespiratory endurance.

Alcohol. Alcohol and exercise do not mix. Alcohol constricts the coronary vessels and may restrict coronary flow during vigorous exercise. Participants should allow at least four hours to elapse between alcohol intake and training. Alcohol consumption followed by exercise could be hazardous.

Regularity of Training. In order for training to be effective, exercise must be performed at regular intervals. Spasmodic exercise may be more detrimental than inactivity. It prevents the gradual conditioning and slow cardiovascular changes necessary for fitness adaptation. Three to four sessions per week are needed for optimal benefits. Fitness can not be stored. It must be continually replenished. Individuals who train at irregualr intervals are constantly starting over, always sore, seldom make observable changes and usually drop-out.

Musculoskeletal Aches and Pains.

Aches and pains in the joints and muscle are usually the result of overtraining. Overtraining for the beginner implies trying to do too much too soon. For the veteran, overtraining occurs when you train too many consecutive days without rest, increase intensity, duration or frequency of training beyond normal capabilities and/or continue to train inspite of signs of illness, injury or fatigue. The body needs rest in order to recover and adapt to the training stimulus. Failure to achieve adequate rest will result in fatigue, injury and/or pain.

Sheehan (1978) believes that resting heart rate can be used as an index of overtraining. He recommends that runners make a habit of recording resting heart rate at least three times per day. The first pulse is taken in bed each morning. The second is taken immediately after training and the third is taken 15-minutes post-exercise. These figures are logged daily and serve as baseline criteria. A morning pulse 10 or more beats per minute higher than the base, indicates that the subject has not completely recovered from the previous day's training. Training should be decreased or suspended until the pulse returns to normal.

Failure to start slowly or observe signs of overtraining will usually result in discomfort or injury sufficient to curtail or limit training. Common sites of pain-injury in runners include feet, ankles, knees, hips and low back. Most problems in these areas can be traced to over-use, weak feet, muscle imbalances and/or poorly designed shoes. The following conditions are frequently observed in runners. A brief discussion of the etiology and recommended corrective-preventive techniques for each is presented.

Shin Splints. Shin splints are pains in the anterior compartment of the lower leg. The exact cause of pain is not known, but is thought to be attributable to microscopic tears of the muscle or pulling of the tendon from the periosteum (bone). Pain is usually present in the front of the leg between the tibia and fibula. Pain increases when you rise-up on the toes, rock-back on the heels or attempt to grip the ground with the toes. Shin splints are most prevelent in beginners whose physical efforts exceed the current capability of the musculature of the legs. Pain usually occurs early in the training routine and is most prevalent following activities requiring vigorous running or jumping on hard surfaces. Stop-and-go activities, such as tennis and racquetball, i.e., sports that require you to run on your toes and make sudden changes of direction, increase the possibility of developing shin splints. Improper shoes have also been linked to anterior lower leg pain. Shoes with low heels poor shock absorption capability and poor foot control are contributors to shin splint

Shin splints can also occur in well-conditioned athletes. These usually occur when the athlete switches to lighter shoes, runs on hard surfaces, increases running speed and/or runs up and down hills. A recent survey by Runner's World indicates that 15 percent of distance runners experience shin splints severe enough to force cessation of training at one time or another. The calf muscles make up approximately four-fifths of the bulk of the lower leg, the anti-gravity muscles on the front of the lower leg make up only one-fifth. Prevention of shin splints requires both the strengthening of the anterior leg muscles and stretching of the posterior calf muscles. Effective exercises for stretching the calf are included in Figure 24. Weak anti-gravity muscles can be strengthened by hanging a five pound weight across the toes as the subject sits erect on the edge of a table (Figure 25). From this position, the subject moves the foot up and down 10-15 times.

The initial concern for individuals with shin splints is to reduce inflammation. This is accomplished by massaging the affected area with ice for approximately 6 minutes after exercise. In addition, you should rest for 2 to 3 days. Most individuals find that rest, aspirin (2 aspririn before and after training), slow running on soft surfaces, strengthening exercises and post-exercise ice massage are effective therapeutic techniques for combating shin splints (Subtonick, 1979).

Tight Calf Muscles and Achille's Pain. Pain in the calf muscle usually occurs as the result of poor running form and inadequate shoes. Individuals who run on their toes keep the calf muscle in almost continuous contraction. With prolonged use, the muscle hypertrophys, shortens and loses flexibility. Calf tightness can also be precipitated by running in shoes with low or worn-down heels, by running farther or faster, and by running up and down hills.

Loss of flexibility in the calf muscle puts additional stress on the Achille's tendon. Sudden stresses and strains at foot strike and take-off are absorbed by the heel cord. Prolonged stress causes the heel cord and/or the sheath covering it to become inflammed (tendinitis). The tendon becomes thicker, tender to touch and painful during walking running.

Achille's tendinitis is prevented and corrected by stretching the calf muscles. Effective exercises for stretching the calf are presented in Figure 24. These exercises should be performed before and after training. Individuals prone to calf tightness might be wise to pause frequently during running or participation in sports and perform the first stretching exercise depicted in Figure 24. Additional precautionary-remedial techniques include the taking of aspirin before and after activity and an ice massage after activity.

FIGURE 24

151

EXERCISES FOR THE ANKLE AND CALF

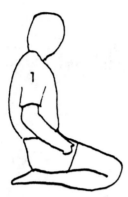

2. Keep rear heel flat.
Slowly move hips
forward. Hold for
20 - 30 seconds each
leg.

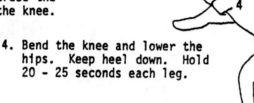

1. Kneel and extend the ankles straight
behind. Do not allow feet to flare out.
A flared-out position may stress the
ligaments on the inside of the knee.
Hold for 15 - 20 seconds.

4. Bend the knee and lower the
hips. Keep heel down. Hold
20 - 25 seconds each leg.

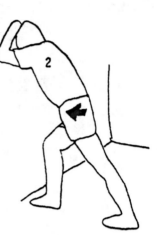

3. Place toes of one foot even to knee
of the other leg. Allow heel of bent
leg to come off the floor. 1/2 inch.
Lower heel while pushing forward on
the thigh with chest and shoulder.
Hold for 10 - 15 seconds each leg.

5. Start from position #2.
Turn the right hip to
the inside and project
the right hip to the
side as you lean your
shoulder in the opposite
direction of your hips.
Hold 20 - 25 seconds
each side.

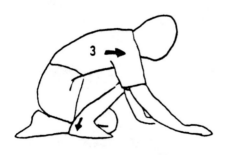

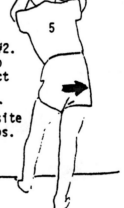

FIGURE 25

REMEDIAL EXERCISE FOR SHIN SPLINTS

Hang a 5 - 10 pound bag over the toes. Lift and hold for 5 seconds. Lower slowly. Repeat 10 - 15 times each leg.

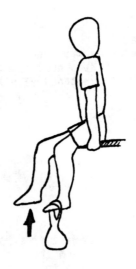

Ankle Strains-Sprains. Strains are injuries to the muscle and/or attachment of the tendon to muscle or tendon to bones. Sprains are injuries to ligaments which attach bone to bone. The ankle joint which consists of 26 bones, tendons and ligaments is a rather unstable joint and is a major site of injury in amateur and professional athletes. Studies suggest that 34 percent of all athletic injuries and 7 percent of all running injuries involve the ankle.

Ankle injuries can involve trauma (stepping in a hole and "turning the ankle."), structural defects (flat feet) or lack of flexibility (plantor faciitis). Prevention and treatment for most ankle injuries are the same. Exercise prior to activity to prevent injury, and ice, elevation and pressure after injury to minimize inflammation. Sample exercises to strengthen the ankle are presented in Figure 24.

Planterfascia and Heel Spur. The biomechanics of running indicates that the heel of the foot should strike the ground first. After heel strike, the force is distributed to the outer border of the foot, the ball of the foot and the toes. After contact, the foot is turned in (pronated), the arch flattened and the thigh rotated inward. The purpose of this motion is to absorb the impact force of the body, which is estimated to be 3 times body weight. Failure to adequately dissipate this force can result in trauma to the soft tissue of the foot, ankle, knee, hip and/or low back.

Lack of flexibility in the muscles of the foot and calf will limit the ability of the ankle to pronate (turn-in) and absorb force. To compensate for this limitation, the arch must flatten farther than normal to help absorb some of the impact force. This action stretches muscles and tendons under the sole of the foot. Prolonged or repeated stress will cause the fascia sheet covering the muscles under the arch to become inflammed (Planterfaciitis) and extremely sore. The site of pain in planterfasciitis is either in the arch or at the attachment of the planterfascia to the bottom of the heel.

Chronic pulling of the planterfascia can cause a heel spur, i.e., an extrusion of bone on the under surface of the heel. Individuals with high, inflexible arches and those who train on hard surfaces, use poor shoes, and drastically increase the intensity and quanity of training are more predisposed to planterfascia and heel spurs.

Prevention consist of stretching exercises (Figure 24) and wearing shoes with a good heel counter, relatively high heel, solid shank and a multi-layered sole. Treatment consists of rest, reduction in work output and running less on the ball of the foot. Runners are encouraged to run every other day on soft surfaces. Taping, heel lifts (.25 to .50 inch of surgical felt or sponge rubber hollowed out like a doughnut), calf stretching exercises, aspirin, heat before and ice after running are recommended ways of coping with planterfascia and heel spurs (Subotnick, 1979). Chronic cases may require a fitting for orthodics. Orthodics should be flexible. Rigid orthodics have been observed to cause or aggravate foot problems.

Morton's Foot. Another major cause of foot pain is Morton's foot, i.e., the second toe is longer than the first or big toe. This condition causes abnormal weight-bearing on the first metatarsal head (base of bone leading from ankle to big toe). The foot contains 5 metatarsal bones, one for each toe which should share weight-bearing evenly. In Morton's foot, the first metatarsal is short. Thus, the second metatarsal receives the bulk of the body's weight. The first not only fails to take its share, but takes it too late. The end result is that the foot pronates or rolls over to the inside. If unchecked, this condition often results in stress fractures of the metatarsals, planterfasciitis, heel spurs, arch and knee pain. These conditions are aggravated and more common in individuals with tight calf muscles.

Individuals with Morton's foot should use shoes with a good control, i.e., a shoe with a good, solid, wide heel and some flexibility, but little compressibility in the sole, and increase the flexibility of the calf and foot. Failure to check the problems associated with Morton's foot could necessitate the purchase of custom designed soft, full-foot orthodics.

Short Leg. The short leg syndrome refers to those foot, leg, knee and low back problems caused by one leg being shorter than the other. Klein (1967) estimates that approximately 50 percent of the population has one leg that is at least .25 inches shorter than the other. The short leg is usually on the dominate side and in some individuals, the shortening is only from the ankle down, i.e., caused by weakness in the foot. Discomfort is usually felt in the longer limb. Correction consists of placing a felt insert, no more than .50 inches in thickness, in the shoe on the short side. Unless symptoms appear, you should not try to correct a short leg.

Knee Injury. Knee injuries are usually the result of impact or trauma or chronic overuse. This discussion will be limited to the latter. Individuals engaged in training often experience knee pain in one of four places; behind the knee cap, outside the knee cap (lateral), inside the knee cap (medial) or below the knee cap.

Runner's knee is a catch-all term for knee cap pain. The knee cap or patella is a sesmoid bone (small extra bone) designed to protect the knee joint. The anterior side of the patella is convex. The posterior side is lined with cartilage and is marked with a lateral and medial facet (Figure 26). These facets articulate with the condyles of the femur and keep the patella in track. Failure of the patella to track evenly causes excess wear on the cartilage covering the patella and femur and the pain associated with "runner's knee." Symtoms of uneven tracking usually progress from tightness around the knee to dull ache and finally pain. In runners, pain is usually mileage related and appears when the participant runs 30 miles per week or more (Subotnick, 1979).

If the stress is continued, the cartilage may soften, crack and give rise to a grinding sensation under the knee cap. This condition is called chondromalacia. With chondromalacia, pain usually occurs when the knee is flexed beyond an angle of 15 degrees. Individuals can usually ride a bicycle with little difficulty, but experience extreme discomfort when ascending or descending hills and stairs. Any pressure on the knee that pushes the patella to the outside or inside causes

FIGURE 26

ANATOMY OF KNEE AND PATELLA *

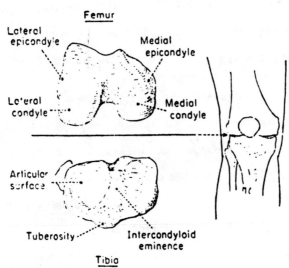

Figure 16-1. Articulating surfaces of knee joint.

* Wells (1971)

excruciating pain. This condition appears to occur more frequently in individuls with flat feet, pronated ankles, leg length discrepancies, tight calves and weak quadriceps. Corrective techniques require strengthening of the quadriceps group, expecially the vastus medialis. Strong anterior thigh muscles keep the patella in track and lessen the chances of developing chondromalacia. Treatment includes rest until pain ceases and then quadricep exercises. Some individuals find that orthodics help prevent-alleviate knee pain. Specific quadricep exercises are illustrated in Figure 27.

Pain on the lateral aspect of the knee, sometimes called iliotibial band syndrome, involves the tensor fascia lata muscle. This muscle is attached to the of the thigh from the hip to just below the knee. The muscle is attached to the tibia (lower leg bone) by a thin tendon band. With over-exertion and fatigue, the muscle tightens and pulls on the tendon which snaps forward over the lateral condyle (protrusion) of the tibia when the knee flexes. The movement of the band causes a snapping or irritation of the tissues and produces a very sharp pain. The iliotibial band can be palpated (felt) while sitting with the leg completely extended by placing your fingers on the outside of the knee. As you flex the leg, the tendon can be felt moving across the tibia. If the band feels tight, snaps and produces pain on knee flexion, iliotibial band syndrome is suggested.

Treatment for this condition includes rest, a reduction in mileage, a decrease in training intensity and an avoidance of hills. Aspirin should be taken 2 to 3 hours before training, an elastic wrap should be worn during activity and ice should be applied after training. Stretching exercises depicted in Figure 28 (Subotnick, 1979). should be done daily.

Pain on the inside of the knee is caused by excess pronation, inward rotation. With excess pronation, the inner border (arch) of the foot collapses and the leg rotates internally causing strain on the inner aspect of the knee. Strain usually involves the bursae of the pes amsrinus, a structure encasing three tendons of the

FIGURE 27

QUADRICEP EXERCISES

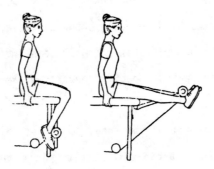

Anterior thigh or quadricep machine

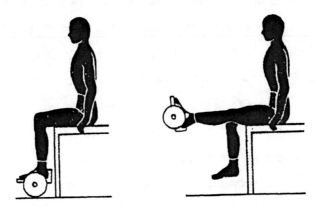

Iron boot exercise

FIGURE 28

STRETCHING EXERCISES FOR ILIOTIBIAL BAND SYNDROME

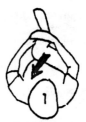

1. Pull knee to chest and then pull it across the body toward the opposite shoulder. Hold for 15 - 20 seconds each leg.

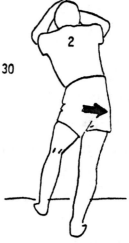

2. Start as is calf stretch. Turn right hip to inside and lean the upper body to the left. Hold for 20 - 30 seconds each side.

hamstrings on the inside of the knee. These tendons rub agaisnt each other or against the underlying soft tissue and bone and cause bursitis, inflammation of the bursa of the knee. Pain on the inner side of the leg usually responds to foot control devices such as orthodics or vargus wedge. Aspirin, ice and rest are also recommended to help reduce inflammation and pain. The self-test for pes bursitis is the presence of rubbing, popping, snapping or pain during knee flexion.

Pain behind the knee is usually due to strain of hamstrings and gastronemius muscles. These muscles become tense with running and are prone to injury when stressed or fatigued. Prevention is the key to avoiding pain behind the knee. Hamstring-gastrocnemius stretching exercises (Figure 29) should be performed daily. In addition, attention should be directed to the task of strengthening the hamstrings. Research indicates that hamstrings must be at least 60 percent as strong as the quadriceps. Individuals who fail to achieve a hamstring-quadricep ratio of at least 60 percent are more prone to hamstring pulls and pain behind the knee.

Hip Pain. Pain in the hip, like pain on the outside of the knee, is due to iliotibial band syndrome. With over-exertion, the tendon of the tensor fascia lata tightens and can snap over the knee joint or over the greater trochanter of the hip and cause bursitis. Treatment for iliotibial band syndrome at the hip is similar to that for iliotibial band syndrome at the knee.

Back Ache. Most cases of back ache are attributable to sciatica or low back pain. Sciatica is inflammation of the sciatic nerve. Inflammation of the sciatic nerve, which originates at the nerve root of the fourth lumbar spine, causes pain to shoot down the back, radiate underneath the buttocks, down the inner-posterior portions of the thigh and down the calf. Pain usually occurs when you straighten the leg from a sitting or supine position.

Sciatica is often related to tight gluteals, tense hamstrings and imbalances between the musculature of the abdomen and low back. Treatment usually involves

FIGURE 29

ABDOMINAL EXERCISES

1. Curl head and shoulders about 6-inches off the floor. Keep chin to chest. Hold for 6-seconds. Relax and repeat 5 - 10 times.

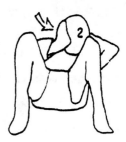

2. Curl head and shoulders off the floor. Gently pull the head and chin toward the left knee. Hold for 6 seconds. Relax and repeat to opposite side. Repeat 5 - 10 times each side.

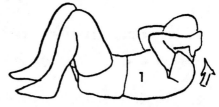

3. Curl head and shoulders off the floor and bring knees to elbows. Hold 6 seconds. Repeat 5 - 10 times.

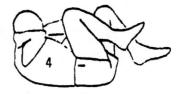

4. Curl head and shoulders off the floor. Gently pull the head and chin toward the left knee. Hold for 6 seconds. Relax. Repeat to the opposite side. Repeat 5 - 10 times each side.

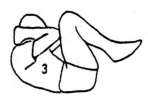

TABLE 32

ABDOMINAL EXERCISES

SIT-UPS

1. Placement. Lie on your back. Bend your knees, place feet parallel to each other on a wall. Cross your arms and hold each elbow with opposite hand.

2. Variation. Exhale, tuck the chin to the chest and lift the head and the upper back, one vertebra at a time off the floor. Shoulders are low, away from ears. Lift with control, lower with control. As with stretching, never jerk.

3. Variation. Begin as in No. 1. Interlace fingers behind head. Exhale, roll head and upper back up as in No. 2. Flex hips and touch the elbows to thighs above the knees. Place toes on wall, lower the upper back, but do not place head to floor. Contract the stomach again, repeating exercise. Begin by doing 2 or 3, work up to 10.

4. Variation. To strengthen the oblique muscles begin as in No. 3 with toes on wall. Flex as in No. 3, but cross the right elbow to touch the left knee, then cross the left elbow to right knee. Release by placing toes on wall, upper back down, head lifted. Repeat as many times as possible without strain, remembering that it's the elbows that cross, not the knees.

stretching of the gluteals, hamstrings and back musculature and development of the abdominal muscles. Effective stretching and strengthening exercises for sciatica are depicted in Figure 16 (Subotnick, 1979).

Low back pain, like sciatica, is due to postural instability, i.e., strength/ flexibility imbalance between the muscles of the abdomen and back and tightness in the gluteal, hamstring and calf musculature. Therapeutic treatment for low back pain consists of tightening the abdominal, flattening the spine and stretching the muscles of the back, gluteals, hamstrings and calves. Specific abdominal exercises are depicted in Figure 30 and Table 32.

Biomechanics of Running.

One of the most critical aspects fo running is the way that the foot contacts the ground. The action of the foot striking the ground and then pushing off propels the runner forward. Most authorities divide the time that the foot is in contact with the ground into 3 phases; (1) heel contact; (2) support and (3) toe off.

At contact, the foot should land on the outer surface of the heel approximately .50 to .75 inch forward of the posterior projection of the heel. Landing on the heel will enable the ankle joint to pronate (turn inward) and absorb some of the shock that occurs when the foot strikes the ground. Estimates suggest that the force of impact on contact for level running is approximately 3 times body weight. The force while running downhill is estimated to be 5 times body weight.

After heel contact, the force is directed to the outside border of the foot, across the arch and finally to the ball of the foot. Shoes should show wear at the outer portion of the heel and under the ball of the foot. As the foot contacts the surface the arch flattens and the foot pronates to absorb shock. When pronation is completed (or almost completed), the knee cap, thigh and hip rotate internally to help abosrb the impact force. Individuals with weak or flat feet tend to over pronate and place excess stress on the longitudinal arch of the foot and inner aspect of the knee. Likewise, a high arched-foot will not give and thus most of the shock is transmitted up the leg and may cause knee, thigh, hip or back problems.

As the weight of the body passes over the support foot, the foot supinates (turns out) and the leg rotates outward. These movements enable the foot to change from a mobile adapter (shock absorber) to a neutral support structure at mid-stance and then a rigid lever at take-off. In the mid-stance position, the bones and joints line up to protect the structural integrity of the arch of the foot. Muscle action is limited and most of the weight is borne by the bones rather than the soft tissue support structures.

At take-off, the weight rolls over the ball of the foot to the toes. This action requires an ample degree of flexibility at the metarsal-tarsal joints (junction of toes and foot). Extreme muscular force is not needed at toe-off because the body's momentum forces it forward and across the metatarsophalangeal joints and phalanges (toes).

When running, the foot should land directly beneath the center of gravity of the body so the body can gently roll over the foot. In other works, the foot should swing forward, then backward and finally land beneath the center of gravity as the body catches up with the foot. Failure to do so causes you to overstride or understride. Runners who overstride place the foot ahead of the center of gravity. This produces a breaking action (slows you down and pushes you back), increases shock and causes excessive heel wear. Runners who understride land on the ball of the foot and place excess stress on the calf muscles and Achille's tendon.

Finally, the feet should contact the ground so that the inner border of each foot should contact a straight line drawn between the feet. Wider stances and those that permit the toes to turn out cause stress on the hips and tend to propel the runner laterally (to the side) with each step. Running with the toes inward (pigeon toed) is counter productive and forces the body to run across itself.

Stride length and stride frequency are related to running speed. Cinematographic analysis indicates that stride frequency increases and stride length decreases as running speed is increased. Likewise, stride length increases and frequency decreases as running speed is reduced. Research suggests that given ample practice, the average individual will determine his own optimal combination of stride length and frequency. Attempts to scientifically improve on self-choice are of limited value.

Arm carry is another important component of good running form. Runners should relax the shoulders, permit a relaxed bend at the elbows and gently cup the hands so the thumb rests gently in the tip of the index finger. The elbows should gently brush the waistband and the forearms should be parallel to the ground. The hands should be carried at waist height, approximately 2 to 3 inches in front of the stomach, and allowed to swing gently away from and across the body. Proper arm swing occurs from the shoulders, not the elbows. The hands should scratch the stomach on the forward swing, but should not cross the midline of the body. On the backswing, the hands should touch tne midline of the hips. Arm movement should be opposite leg movement, i.e., the right arm comes forward as the right leg is extended and vice-versa.

Extraneous movements and tense arm carry uses energy and are inefficient Some runners, especially women, tend to swing their arms from side to side. This action dissipates energy sideways, causes excessive rotation of the trunk and works against the forward thrust of the legs. The final consideration in running form is head carry. The head should be carried high. Failure to do so, restricts air flow, causes the shoulders to slump and tilts the center gravity forward.

Warm-Up and Cool Down.

Most training sessions consist of three essential parts: (1) warm-up; (2) vigorous conditioning and (3) cool-down. Each segment is essential for safe, effective training.

Prior to each workout, participants should engage in a 5-10 minutes of exercise designed to help prepare them physically and mentally for the upcoming exertion. Two classifications of warm-up exist; specific and general. Specific warm-up involves practicing or rehearsing the specific event or skill a few times prior to competitive performance. Shooting free throws and taking batting practice are of specific warm-up. General warm-up includes exercise unrelated to the competitive event. Calisthenics and stretching exercises are examples of general warm-up.

Most individuals involved in physical fitness programs utilize general warm-up exercises. Warm-up prepares the body for the upcoming workout and protects the body against unnecessary injuries and muscle soreness. In addition, it stimulates the heart and lungs, increases circulation and raises body temperature. A thorough warm-up gradually stretches the muscles and tendons and prepares them for forceful contrations.

Research (Garfield, 1977) suggests that the most important function of warm-up is increasing body temperature. Cellular metabolism is temperature dependent. Most metabolic (chemical) reactions are speeded up when body temperature is increased. Astrand and Rodahl (1970) suggests that metabolic rate will increase 10-13 percent for each degree increase in body temperature. As temperature increases, nerve impulses travel faster and the muscles become better prepared for increased exertion. Muscles contract, relax and recover faster following active warm-up. Increases in internal temperature cause the blood vessels in the muscles to dilate which increases the flow of nutrients to the muscles and facilitates the flow of waste products away from the muscles.

With warm-up, the hemoglobin (oxygen-carrying compound in the blood) and myoglobin (oxygen storing compound inside the muscle) release more oxygen. Blood flow through the lungs is increased, which enhances the exchange of oxygen and carbon dioxide in the alveoli and increases the efficiency of the cardiorespiratory system. During maximal effort, aerobic capacity is improved following warm-up.

For most individuals, warm-up exercises should be performed for at least 10-15 minutes. Data (Astrand and Radahl, 1970) suggest that warm-up bouts within this range will elevate body temperature by 1-2 degrees F. A crude indices of sufficient warm-up is the presence of perspiration. Participants should carefully monitor their efforts.

Insufficient warm-up may not raise the body temperature sufficiently and too much can cause fatigue. Examples of active, general warm-up routines for specific activities are presented in Figures 30 to 37 .

Following sufficient warm-up, participants are prepared to perform the main conditioning segment of the workout. Aerobic activities such as jogging, walking, cycling and swimming are recommended. Activities that are continuous and rhythmic should be emphasized. On alternate days, participants may elect to use sports such as racquetball, handball, tennis or basketball as their principle form of training. A discussion of these activities is presented in Chapter 4.

In most workouts, the intensity of effort should be sufficient to raise the heart rate to approximately 75 percent of maximum (target heart rate). Peak efforts should not exceed 90 percent of maximum heart rate. Initial efforts should be sustained for approximately 20 minutes. With time and adaptation, the duration of effort can be gradually extended. A safe rule of thumb limits progress to 10 percent per week. A beginner who exercises for 20 minutes the first week should be able to safely sustain similar effort for 22 minutes (20 minutes X 110%) the second week.

Individuals who engage in strength training, should do so after aerobic activities are completed or on alternate days. Weight training can cause local muscular fatigue and restrict the main conditioning segment of the workout (running, cycling, etc.) and, therefore, should be performed after aerobic exercises. Strength training conducted on the same day as aerobic training should be performed following warm-up exercises designed for this purpose (Figure 30). Warm-up exercises for other forms of training are presented in Figures 31 to 36.

The cool down is the tapering-off period after completion of the main workout. It is best accomplished by a continuation of the training activity at a lowered intensity In other words, keep moving. Walking is the most common method of gradually diminishing intensity. Slow jogging is another effective cool down procedure.

Cool down activities prevent the blood from pooling in the extremeties and legs by allowing the muscles to assist in pumping blood from the extremeties to the heart.

FIGURE 30

WARM-UP EXERCISES FOR STRENGTH TRAINING

1. Gently pull elbow behind the head. Hold 10 - 15 seconds.

2. Interlace fingers, turn palms up above the head and straighten the arms. Hold 10 - 15 seconds. Repeat 3 - 5 times.

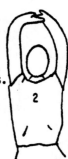

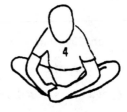

3. Keep rear heel flat. Slowly move hips forward. Hold for 20 - 30 seconds each leg.

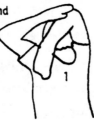

4. Place soles of feet together and grasp toes. Gently bend forward from the hips. Hold 30 - 40 seconds

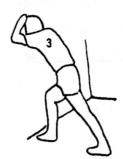

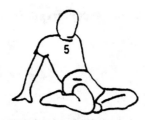

5. Sit with the right leg bent, heel to the outside of the right hip. Left leg is bent and sole of the foot is next to inside of right thigh. Keep right foot straight and lean backwards. Hold for 20 - 30 seconds each leg.

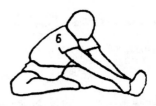

6. Straighten right leg. Place sole of left foot against inside of right thigh. Bend forward at hips and hold for 20 seconds. Bend farther and hold for 20 seconds. Repeat for left leg.

FIGURE 31   169

WARM-UP EXERCISES FOR BASKETBALL

1. Fold arms over head.
   Bend to right. Hold
   for 20 - 30 seconds
   each side.

2. Interlace
   fingers, turn
   palms up above
   the head and
   straighten the
   arms. Hold 10 -
   15 seconds.
   Repeat 3 - 5
   times.

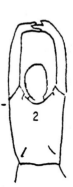

3. Place soles of feet
   together and grasp toes!
   Gently bend forward from
   the hips. Hold 30 - 40
   seconds.

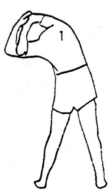

4. Cross leg over the knee and pull
   bottom leg toward
   the floor.
   Hold for 20 -
   30 seconds each
   side.

5. Pull knee to chest and hold for 15
   seconds each leg. Keep back and
   neck flat.

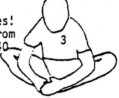

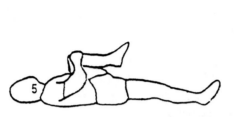

6. Kneel on both knees. Move one leg
   forward until knee is over the ankle.
   Lower hip and hold for 30 seconds
   each leg.

170

FIGURE 31 contd.

7. Sit with the right leg bent, heel to the outside of the right hip. Left leg is bent and sole of the foot is next to inside of right thigh. Keep right foot straight and lean backwards. Hold for 20 - 30 seconds each leg.

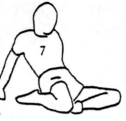

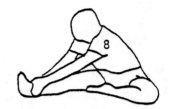

8. Straighten right leg. Place sole of left foot against inside of right thigh. Bend forward at hips and hold for 20 seconds. Bend farther and hold for 20 seconds. Repeat for left leg.

9. On all fours, fingers facing back. Move weight toward hips. Keep palms flat. Hold 10 - 15 seconds.

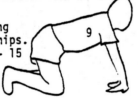

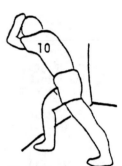

10. Keep rear heel flat. Slowly move hips forward. Hold for 20 - 30 seconds each leg.

FIGURE 32

WARM-UP EXERCISES FOR CYCLING

1. Cross leg over the knee and pull bottom leg toward the floor. Hold for 20 - 30 seconds each side.

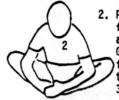

2. Place soles of feet together and grasp toes. Gently bend forward from the hips. Hold 30 - 40 seconds.

3. Sit with right leg straight. Bend left leg. Cross left foot over and rest it to outside of right knee. Rest right elbow on outside of upper left thigh. Look over left shoulder and rotate upper body to the left. Hold 10 - 15 seconds.

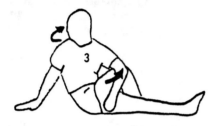

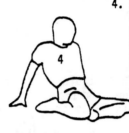

4. Sit with right leg bent, heel to the outside of the right hip. Left leg is bent and sole of the foot is next to inside of right thigh. Keep right foot straight and lean backwards. Hold 20 - 30 seconds each leg.

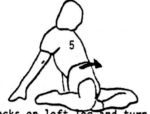

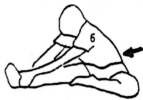

5. Tighten buttocks on left leg and turn hips to right. Hold 5 - 10 seconds each leg.

6. Straighten right leg. Place sole of left foot against inside of right thigh. Bend forward at hips and hold for 20 seconds. Bend farther and hold for 20 seconds. Repeat for left leg.

FIGURE 32 contd.

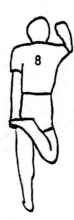

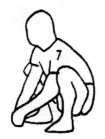

7. Squat down, feet flat, toes out 10 - 15 degrees and heels 4 - 12 inches apart. Hold 30 seconds

8. Hold right foot with left hand and pull heel to buttocks. Hold 20 - 30 seconds each leg.

9. Place ball of foot on table or fence. Bend knee and move hips forward. Hold 30 seconds each leg.

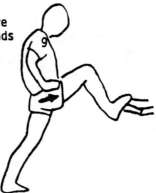

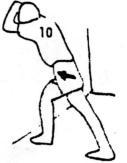

10. Keep rear heel flat. Slowly move hips forward. Hold for 20 - 30 seconds each leg.

FIGURE 33

WARM-UP EXERCISES FOR GOLF

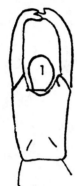

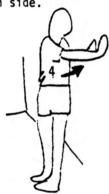

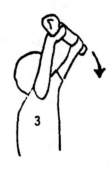

2. Fold arms over head. Bend to right. Hold for 20 - 30 seconds each side.

1. Interlace fingers, turn palms up above the head and straighten the arms. Hold 10 - 15 seconds.

3. Grasp towel near ends. Lift over head and lower behind the back. Hold 10 - 20 seconds.

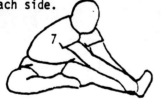

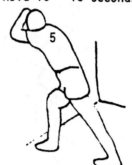

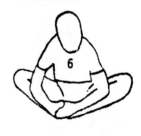

4. Stand 12 - 24 inches away from fence or wall. Turn until hands touch wall at shoulder height. Return and hold 20 seconds each side.

5. Keep rear heel flat. Slowly move hips forward. Hold 20 - 30 seconds each leg.

6. Place soles feet togethe and grasp to Gently bend forward from the hips. Hold 30 - 40 seconds.

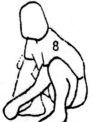

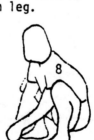

7. Straighten right leg. Place sole of left foot against inside of right thigh. Bend forward at hips and hold for 20 seconds. Bend farther and hold for 20 seconds. Repeat for left leg.

8. Squat down, feet flat, toes out 10 - 15 degrees and heels 4 - 12 inches apart. Hold 30 seconds.

FIGURE 34

WARM-UP EXERCISES FOR TENNIS, RACQUETBALL AND HANDBALL

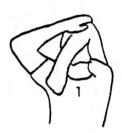

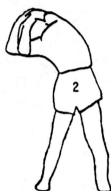

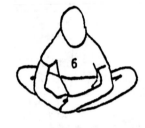

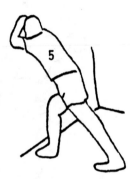

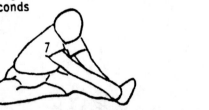

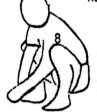

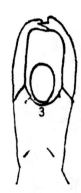

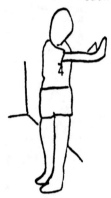

1. Gently pull elbow behind the head. Hold 10 - 15 seconds.

2. Fold arms over head. Bend to right. Hold for 20 -30 seconds each side.

3. Interlace fingers, turn palms up above the head and straighten the arms. Hold 10 - 15 seconds.

4. Stand 12 - 24 inches away from fence or wall. Turn until hands touch wall at shoulder height. Return, hold 20 seconds each side.

5. Keep rear heel flat. Slowly move hips forward. Hold 20 - 30 seconds each side.

6. Place soles of feet together and grasp toes. Gently bend forward from hips. Hold 30 - 40 seconds

7. Straighten right leg. Place sole of left foot against inside of right thigh. Bend forward at hips and hold for 20 seconds. Bend farther and hold for 20 seconds. Repeat for left leg.

8. Squat down, feet flat, toes out 10 - 15 degrees and heels 4 - 12 inches apart. Hold 30 seconds.

FIGURE 34 contd.

9. Place toes of one foot even to knee of the other leg. Allow heel of bent leg to come off the floor 1/2 inch. Lower heel while pushing forward on the thigh with chest and shoulder. Hold 10 - 15 seconds each leg.

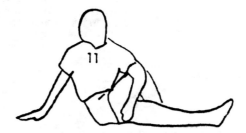

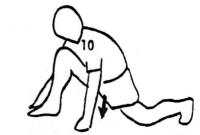

11. Sit with right leg straight. Bend left leg. Cross left foot over and rest it to outside of right knee. Rest right elbow on outside of upper left thigh. Look over left shoulder and rotate upper body to the left. Hold 10 - 15 seconds each side.

10. Kneel down. Bend forward and place weight over front foot. Slowly extend rear leg and push groin toward the floor. Hold 20 - 30 seconds each leg.

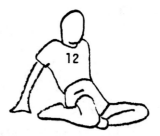

13. Cross leg over the knee and pull bottom leg toward the floor. Hold for 20 - 30 seconds each side.

12. Sit with right leg bent, heel to the outside of the right hip. Left leg is bent and sole of the foot is next to inside of right thigh. Keep right foot straight and lean backwards. Hold 20 - 30 seconds each leg.

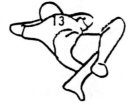

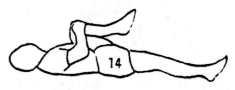

14. Pull knee to chest and hold for 15 seconds each leg. Keep back and neck flat.

FIGURE 35

WARM-UP EXERCISES FOR RUNNING

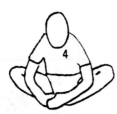

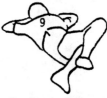

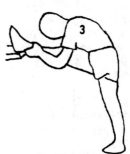

1. Keep rear heel flat. Slowly move hips forward. Hold 20 - 30 seconds each side.

2. Bend the knee and lower the hips. Keep heel down. Hold 20 - 25 seconds each leg.

3. Place heel on table. Bend support knee 1 - 2 inches and lower hips so they are parallel. Bend forward at the waist and hold 10 - 15 seconds. Relax and increase stretch.

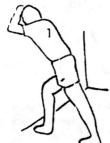

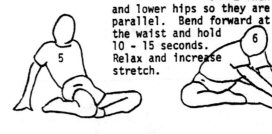

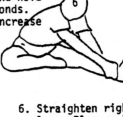

4. Place soles of feet together and grasp toes. Gently bend forward from hips. Hold 30 - 40 seconds.

5. Sit with right leg bent, heel to outside of right hip. Left leg is bent and sole of foot is next to inside of right thigh. Keep right foot straight and lean backwards. Hold 20 - 30 seconds each leg.

6. Straighten right leg. Place sole of left foot against inside of right thigh. Bend forward at hips and hold for 20 seconds. Bend farther and hold.

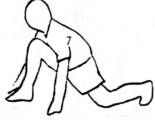

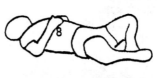

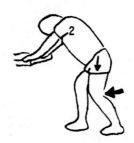

7. Kneel down. Bend forward and place weight over front foot. Slowly extend rear leg and push groin toward floor. Hold 20 - 30 seconds each leg.

8. Place soles of feet together. Relax and hold 20 - 30 seconds.

9. Cross leg over knee and pull bottom leg toward the floor. Hold 20 - 30 seconds each side.

DO BEFORE AND AFTER RUNNING

FIGURE 36

STRETCHING EXERCISES FOR WORK AND/OR TRAVEL

1. Tighten quadriceps and relax hamstrings with knees bent. Hold 20 - 30 seconds.

2. Keep rear heel flat. Slowly move hips forward. Hold 20 - 30 seconds each leg.

3. With knees slightly bent, relax arms and neck and bend forward at the waist. Hold 20 - 30 seconds.

4. Squat down, feet flat, toes out 10 - 15 degrees and heels 4 - 12 inches apart. Hold 30 seconds.

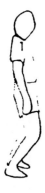 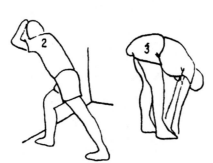 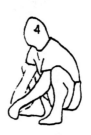

5. Place both hands shoulder-width apart on a ledge and let upper body drop down as you bend your knees 1 - 2 inches. Hold 15 - 20 seconds

6. Interlace fingers, turn palms up above the head and straight the arms. Hold 10 - 15 seconds.

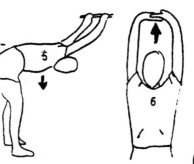

8. Slowly roll head in a full circle. Keep back straight and hold 5 - 10 seconds at each point in circle.

9. Pull opposite heel to buttocks with opposite hand Hold 20 - 30 seconds each leg.

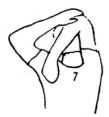 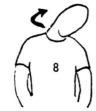

7. Gently pull elbow behind the head. Hold 10 - 15 seconds.

Slow rhythmic activity rids the muscles of fluid build-up and metabolic wastes associated with exercise. These wastes are thought to be major contributors to post-exercise muscle soreness. Most authorities recommend that cool down activities be continued for 3-5 minutes. Cooper (1978) contends that a post-exercise heart rate of less than 120 beats per minute is indicative of adequate cool down.

CHAPTER 8
GETTING STARTED

The purpose of this chapter is to help you get started on a safe, effective physical fitness program. Specific topics to be discussed include: (1) how to determine your current level of fitness; (2) how to design an effective conditioning program and (3) how to implement a personalized fitness program.

Several tests of the various components of physical fitness will be presented. The purpose of these tests is to determine initial physical fitness status. Results from these tests will serve as the basis for preparing a safe, personalized exercise prescription. In addition, test results will be used as a baseline for future comparisons and motivationalpurposes. The development of a personalized exercise prescription will ensure that the effort required in training is within the capacity limits of the participant.

Normative data for adult males and females will be presented for each fitness test. These norms will enable you to determine your status and identify strengths and weaknesses. Also included are sample conditioning programs with recommended rates of progression. Once an individual is tested, he can assess his status (normative data), refer to the various conditioning programs to determine his starting point and then follow the progressions outlined.

Tests of Cardiorespiratory Endurance.

As indicated in Chapter 4, clinical tests of cardiorespiratory endurance are usually performed on either a motor-driven treadmill or bicycle ergometer. Test results are expressed in terms of maximal oxygen uptake ($ml\ O_2/min$ or $ml\ O_2/Kg/min$), i.e., the volume of oxygen taken in and utilized per minute. Normative data have been established for age and sex and are depicted in Table 6. If access to clinical tests are not available and no contraindications exist, field tests can be used to estimate aerobic capacity.

The simplest field tests of aerobic capacity are the 12-minute run and 1.5-mile run. In the 12-minute run test, the runner is asked to cover as much distance as possible in 12 minutes. The objective of the 1.5-mile test is to run or run-walk 1.5 miles as fast as possible. Research (Cooper,1978) indicates that the correlation between these tests and clinical tests of aerobic capacity is high (.85-.90). After completing either test, you can compare the results with data in Table 6, 7, or 8, estimate your VO_2 max and determine your fitness classification.

Once initial status is determined, you can prepare an exercise prescription for aerobic training. Individuals who choose to walk and/or jog as their principle mode of training should consult Tables 11 and 12. If test results indicate that aerobic capacity is poor, participants are encouraged to begin walking at week 1 (Table 11). Heart rate should be monitored at 3-5 minute intervals. If heart rate is consistently below threshold (75 percent of age adjusted maximum) and you are not fatigued, you should move up one level at the next workout. Determination of the initial training intensity sometimes requires trial and error. Most individuals can determine the work load that will produce a target heart rate in 1 to 2 sessions. Once the initial workload is established, you should follow the program as outlined.

Individuals who can be classified as being in fair or better condition can choose jogging or walking-jogging as their principle mode of training. The beginning program outlined in Table 12 has been observed to be effective for adults of all ages. If results indicate that you are borderline fair, use the jog-walk routine designed for week 1. Record heart rate after jogging at 3 to 5 minute intervals. If the rate is consistently below threshold, move up one level for the next workout. Repeat the above procedure until a routine is established that will consistently elicit a threshold heart rate.

Do not become discouraged if you fail to elicit a threshold heart rate the first or second time out. There exists some trial and error in selecting the appropriate training routine. For beginners, it is safer to underestimate than overestimate potential. Take your time. Do not try to jump several levels at a time. You are training for the rest of your life. Be patient. Try to enjoy the activity.

If you are classified as being in good or better condition, you can elect to enter the Table at a higher level. The information in Table 33 offers an alternative to the program in Table 12. Table 33 depicts the energy cost (ml O_2/Kg/min) for running a mile at various time intervals, e.g., 6-, 8- or 10-minute mile pace. An individual with a maximum oxygen uptake of 45 ml O_2/Kg/min could refer to this Table and see that the typical individual with a VO_2 max of 45 ml/Kg/min has the capacity to run a mile in approximately 8 minutes. Moving over 1 or 2 columns, the appropriate 1-mile paces for training at 75 and 85 percent of aerobic capacity (upper and lower threshold limits) are given. Individuals who do not like to interrupt their training to check heart rate usually find the information in this Table helpful in choosing and maintaining an optimal level of training. An individual tested and observed to have a VO_2 max of 38.5 ml O_2/Kg/min can be classified as being in fair condition. Inspection of Table 33 indicates that an aerobic capacity of 38.5 ml/Kg/min should permit the subject to run at a 10-minute mile pace. Safe training should occur at speeds between 11:45 and 10:45 mile pace (75 and 85 percent of aerobic capacity).

Individuals who use running as their only means of aerobic conditioning should run at least 20 minutes per day, 3 times per week. Progressions should follow the outline presented in previous paragraphs. Those who seek variety should select from activities such as swimming, cycling, tennis, racquetball, handball and basketball. It is the opinion of this writer, that jogging should be the central theme in most conditioning programs. Alternate activities should be used to minimize boredom and accommodate competitive drives.

Swimming is an excellent means of developing cardiovascular fitness. Specific advantages and limitations to swim training are discussed in Chapter 4. Beginning swimmers are encouraged to use a swim and walk technique during initial training sessions. That is, they should swim one length of the pool, climb out and walk back

TABLE 33

AEROBIC TRAINING PROGRAM BASED ON VO_2 MAX

1-Mile Time (min:sec)	Energy Lost (ml/kg/min)	Pace Time in Miles/Minutes 75%	Pace Time in Miles/Minutes 85%
4:00	77.8	5:30	4:45
4:15	72.7	5:45	5:00
4:30	68.1	6:00	5:15
4:45	64.0	6:15	5:30
5:00	61.6	6:30	5:45
5:15	59.4	6:45	6:00
5:30	57.5	7:00	6:15
5:45	55.7	7:15	6:30
6:00	54.1	7:30	6:45
6:15	52.5	8:00	7:00
6:30	51.1	8:15	7:15
6:45	49.8	8:30	7:30
7:00	48.6	8:45	7:45
7:15	47.4	9:00	8:00
7:30	46.3	9:15	8:15
7:45	45.3	9:30	8:30
8:00	44.3	9:45	8:45
8:15	43.4	10:00	9:00
8:30	42.5	10:15	9:15
8:45	41.7	10:30	9:30
9:00	40.9	10:45	9:45
9:15	40.2	11:00	10:00
9:30	39.5	11:15	10:15
9:45	38.8	11:30	10:30
10:00	38.2	11:45	10:45
10:10	37.6	12:00	11:00
10:30	37.0	12:15	11:15
10:45	36.4	12:30	11:30
11:00	35.9	12:45	11:45
11:15	35.4	13:00	12:00
11:30	34.9	13:15	12:15
11:45	34.4	13:30	12:30
12:00	33.9	13:45	12:45

to the starting point. This procedure is similar to the walk-jog program and should be repeated until 10 laps (10 sets) are swam (approximately 10 minutes). You should try to add 2 laps (sets) per day until you can complete 20 laps (sets) per session. At this time, enter Stage 2 and swim two laps (down and back) before walking Eight sets (16 laps) should be completed on day one. Each succeeding day you should add 2 sets (4 laps) until you reach 20 sets (40 laps).

During Stage 3, swim 3 laps before walking. Six sets (18 laps) are swam initially with 2 sets added daily. The goal for this Stage is 15 sets (30 laps). In Stage 4, 4 laps are swam before walking. Initial workouts require 4 sets (16 laps). Progression is 2 sets per day until you reach 16 sets (32 laps). In each Stage, periodically check your heart rate at the completion of a lap to ensure that you are working near the threshold level (Table 34).

Once you are able to achieve Stage 4, you can choose to swim continuously or continue the swim-walk program. Continuous swimmers should swim 16 to 32 laps (.50 mile). Interval swimmers should use a 4:1 swim-walk ratio and complete at least 16 laps. Estimates indicate that 100 yards of swimming equals 400 yards of running. Thus, 2 miles of jogging is equivalent to approximately .50 mile of swimming.

Bicycling and stationary cycling are both good sources of aerobic conditioning provided the intensity is at least threshold level. Individuals using stationary cycling should use the 5-stage program outlined in Table 35.

Bicycle riders are encouraged to use a 5-step interval program similar to that recommended for stationary cycling. Participants should alternate periods of fast and slow cycling. The energy cost of cycling is approximately 1/3 that in running. You have to cycle approximately twice as fast as you would jog in order to achieve the same heart rate. The following program permits (Table 36) a gradual build-up to continuous cycling. At Stage 5, you can elect to cycle continuously and/or cycle one mile at a reduced speed every 5 miles.

A sample 13-week rope-skipping routine is presented in Table 37. The routines are designed to gradually progress the beginner from brief to continuous skipping.

TABLE 34

BEGINNING SWIMMING PROGRAM

Stage	Swim (laps)	Walk (laps)	Sets	Total Laps	Progression (sets/day)	Goal (laps/day)
1	1	1	10	10	2	20
2	2	1	8	16	2	40
3	3	1	6	18	2	30
4	4	1	4	16	2	32

TABLE 35

BEGINNING STATIONARY CYCLING PROGRAM

Stage	Pedaling Time (min)	Rest Time (min)	Sets (#day)	Progression (sets/day)	Training Goal (Total Sets)	Time (min)
1	2	:30	5	1	8	12-20
2	3	:30	5	1	8	17-28
3	4	:30	4	1	8	18-28
4	5	:30	4	1	8	20-36
5	20-40					20-40

TABLE 36
BEGINNING CYCLING PROGRAM

Stage	Fast Cycling Distance (miles)	Speed (mph)	Time (min)	Slow Cycling Distance (miles)	Time (min)	Speed (mph)	Sets (#/day)	Progression Training (sets/day)	Total sets	Time (min)
1	1	12	5	.25	2	6	5	1	8	5
2	1	15	4	.25	2	6	5	1	10	5
3	1.5	15	6	.25	3	6	5	1	10	6
4	2	15	8	.25	3	6	5	1	10	10
5	10-20	12.-15								10

TABLE 37

ROPE SKIPPING PROGRAM (80 RPM)

Week	Jump (min:sec)	Rest (sec)	Sets	Total Jumping Time (min)
1	:10	10	12	2
2	:15	10	12	3
3	:30	10	12	6
4	1:	15	12	12
5	2 :	30	10	20
6	3 :	30	7	21
7	4 :	30	5	20
8	5 :	30	4	20
9	6 :	30	4	24
10	7 :	60	4	28
11	8 :	60	4	32
12	9 :	60	4	36
13	10 :	120	3	30

Rope speeds of 80 turns (80 rpm) are recommended for each stage. Training heart rate should be at least 75 percent of maximum.

Team and racquet sports such as basketball, tennis, racquetball and handball will effectively increase aerobic fitness if played regularly at high intensity and for sustained periods of time. Research by Cooper (1977), indicates that beginners must play 25-40 minutes per day at least 3 times per week for 6 weeks in order to affect fitness. Thereafter, participants must play 30-60 minutes per day, 4 times per week.

Strength Training.

Strength training is perhaps the second most important portion of the total conditioning program. A variety of techniques are available, e.g., free-weights, Nautilus, Universal Gym, Dyna-Cam, Mini-Gym, isometrics, etc. The advantages/limitations of each of these methods are discussed in Chapter 3.

The most important aspect of strength training is the selection of appropriate training load(s) (intensity). Load selection is usually based on results of initial strength testing and/or body weight. While strength testing yields more accurate data, a number of individuals prefer to estimate intensity from body weight. These estimates are quick and require less physical effort than testing. The procedures for estimating starting loads from body weight are presented in Table 4.

Muscular strength can be assessed clinically or with field tests. Clinical tests require trained personnel and expensive equipment such as Cybex, cable tensiometers, strain gauges, etc. Field testing usually involves determining maximum strength (1-RM) for given lifts. Test procedures for determining one-repetition maximum (1-RM) require some degree of trial and error and are as follows:

(1) Start with a weight that you can lift comfortably.

(2) Add weight and repeat the lift.

(3) If the weight can be lifted more than one time, continue to add weight until the weight can be lifted correctly only one time (1-RM).

Normative 1-RM data for males and females have been determined by Pollock, et al (1977) and are presented in Table 38. Initial training loads should be equivalent to 70 to 85 percent of the 1-RM for each lift. Training should be performed 3 times per week on alternate days. For the first week, subjects should perform 1 set of each lift with a load equal to 75 percent of the 1-RM. Ten repetitions (10-RM) of each lift should be performed.

During the second week, 10 pounds should be added to each lift and one set of each exercise should be performed with this 10-RM load. Upon completion of the first set, an additional 10 pounds should be added to each lift and 6 (6-RM) to 8 (8-RM) repetitions of each lift performed. Additional weight should be added at anytime that you can perform 12 or more repetitions of a given lift with the existing 10-RM load.

After 6 weeks, you may wish to add a third set of each exercise. This is accomplished by adding 10 pounds to the current 8-RM load. The new workout becomes 3 sets with: (1) 10-RM; (2) 8-RM and (3) 6-RM load. As strength increases, the 10-RM becomes the new 8-RM and the 8-RM becomes the new 6-RM.

Abdominal strength is best enhanced by doing isometric or conventional, bent-knee sit-ups. With isometric sit-ups, the fingers are interlaced behind the head or folded across the chest. The exercise is performed by tightening the stomach and curling the head and shoulders 6 to 8 inches off the floor. This position is held for 6 seconds. Ten repetitions should be performed daily during the first week. Each week you should add 10-sit-ups until a total of 40 isometric sit-ups are performed At this point, you should observe the following routine:

(1) 10, 6-second isometric sit-ups

(2) 10, 2-part isometric sit-ups. Curl the head and shoulders up for 6 seconds Then, bring the knees to the elbows and hold for 6-seconds.

(3) 10, V-situps. Simultaneously bring the knees and elbows up to touch. Hold for 6-seconds.

(4) 10, pump sit-ups. Curl the head and shoulder up. Bring the right knee up, twist the body and touch the right knee to the left elbow while simul-

TABLE 38

NORMATIVE 1-RM DATA[a, b, *]

Body Weight	Bench Press		Standing Press		Curl		Leg Press	
(lb)	Male	Female	Male	Female	Male	Female	Male	Female
80	80	56	53	37	40	28	160	112
100	100	70	67	47	50	35	200	140
120	120	84	80	56	60	42	240	168
140	140	98	93	65	70	49	280	196
160	160	112	107	75	80	56	320	224
180	180	126	120	84	90	63	360	252
200	200	140	133	93	100	70	400	280
220	220	154	147	103	110	77	440	308
240	240	168	160	112	120	84	480	336

[a] Data collected on Universal Gym apparatus. Information collected on other apparatus could modify results.

[b] Data expressed in pounds.

*Pollock, et al (1977)

taneously extending the left leg out straight. Without lowering the trunk or legs, repeat to opposite side and do 10 total touches before resting.

(5) 10, Yoga sit-ups (Table 32).

This routine will effectively increase abdominal strength and reduce waist girth. The Yoga sit-ups are designed to tighten the stomach and strengthen the oblique muscle

Conventional sit-ups are performed with the knees bent and fingers interlaced behind the head. Care must be exercised to avoid throwing the elbows forward and/or raising and dropping the hips. These actions use the momentum of the body segments (momentum = mass X velocity) to overcome the inertia (resistance to movement) of the trunk. The end result is that the trunk is thrust forward with minimum involvement of the abdominal muscles. Sit-ups performed on an inclined board usually require muscular action of the anterior leg muscles (shin) and involve a considerable amount of bouncing and arm throwing. Thus, they are often less effective than the aforementioned isometric and Yoga sit-ups.

The routine presented in Table 38 is suggested for those who prefer to use bent-knee sit-ups.

Chin-ups.

Chin-ups are performed with the palms facing the body. This hand position ensures maximum utilization of the biceps brachii muscle which flexes and supinates (turns the palm up) the forearm. The palms forward grip tends to twist the hand off the bar as the forearm flexes and supinates.

Chin-up performance is weight dependent. Heavy individuals are handicapped and usually perform fewer chin-ups than lighter individuals. Individuals who can not do one chin-up should start with an isometric program. This approach requires the subject to stand on a ladder or stool so that the chin is above the chinning bar. Using the reverse grip, the subject steps off the support and holds the chin over the bar for as long as possible. Work rest intervals of 5:30 seconds should

TABLE 35

SIT-UP PROGRAM

| Week | SETS | | | Total (sit-ups) |
	1 (sit-ups)	2 (sit-ups)	3 (sit-ups)	
1	10	10	10	30
2	20	10	10	40
3	30	10	10	50
4	40	10	10	60
5	50	10		60
6	60			

TABLE 40
CHINS-YOYO PROCEDURE

---

(1) Using a ladder or stool place the chin over the bar.

(2) Hold for 6 seconds.

(3) Lower body until eyes are even with bar and hold for 6 seconds.

(4) Raise body to starting position and hold for 6 seconds.

(5) Rest for 30-60 seconds.

(6) Repeat steps 1-5 at least 5 times.

(7) Each week hold., lower and raise the body one additional time before resting.

(8) When you can yo-yo 5 times without rest, proceed to the chinning program presented in Table 40.

TABLE 41

CHINNING PROGRAM

| Week | SETS | | | Total Chins |
	1 Chins	2 Chins	3 Chins	
1	1	1	1	3
2	2	1	1	4
3	3	1	1	5
4	4	1	1	6
5	5	1	1	7
6	6	1	1	8
7	7	1	1	9
8	8	1	1	10
9	9	1	0	10
10	10	0	0	10

be used by very weak individuals. Repetitions should be continued until you have hung from the bar for at least 60 total seconds. Once you can hang for 60 continuous seconds, switch to the yo-yo procedure described in Table 40.

Flexibility.

Flexibility is specific to each joint. Thus, no tests of general body flexibility exist. Two reliable and often used tests of flexibility are the sit-and-reach test and the trunk extension test. The sit-and-reach test assesses the flexibility of the hamstrings and buttocks muscles and the trunk extension test measures the range of motion in the low back region. The following procedures are recommended for the sit-and-reach test:

(1) Sit with legs extended directly in front, knees extended and pressed against the floor.

(2) Place the soles of the feet against a box to which is attached a yardstick. The 14-inch mark on the yardstick is placed at the near edge of the box (junction of foot and box).

(3) Place the index fingers of both hands together and slowly reach as far forward as possible. Keep the knees in contact with the floor. Do not jerk or bounce.

(4) Note and record the distance reached on the yardstick.

(5) Consult standards in Table 42 to determine status.

Procedures for the trunk extension test are as follows:

(1) Lie prone on the floor with partner holding the buttocks and legs.

(2) Interlace fingers behind the head.

(3) Slowly raise the head and trunk from the floor as far as possible.

(4) Hold for 3-5 seconds.

(5) Record distance from floor to chin.

(6) Consult standards in Table 42 to determine status.

TABLE 42

FLEXIBILITY NORMS*

	Sit and Reach	Trunk Extension
Excellent	22 in. or greater	16 in. or greater
Good	19-21 inch	13-15 inch
Average	14-18 inch	10-12 inch
Fair	12-13 inch	8-9 inch
Poor	11 inch or less	7 inch or less

* From Health Improvement Program. National Athletic Health Institute. Inglewood, CA.

Since flexibility is specific to each joint, different stretching exercises are recommended for different activities/sports. The following routines are designed for use in the morning, during work, before training, after training, during travel, before bed and for relief of low back tension. Each routine is simple, requires little time and effort and requires no special clothing. Each stretch should be repeated 3-5 times and should be held for 10-20 seconds. Stretching should be relaxed and should follow guidelines outlined in Chapter 6.

Morning Stretching Exercises (upon rising) - Figure 17.

Stretching Exercises During Work (relieve tension) - Figure 38.

Stretching Exercises Before Training:

    (1) Running, Walking and Cycling - Figures 32 and 35.
    (2) Tennis/Racquet Sports - Figure 34.
    (3) Strength Training - Figure 30.

Stretching Exercises After Training - Figure 35.

Stretching Exercises During Travel - Figure 36.

Stretching Exercise Before Bed-Time - Figure 37.

Stretching Exercises for Relief of Low Back Tension - Figure 16.

Body Composition.

Body composition is assessed to determine nutritional status. Individuals can be measured and body density, relative and absolute fat and lean body weight (bone and muscle) determined. On the basis of these results, individuals can be classified with respect to degree of fatness and an accurate estimate of ideal body weight can be made.

Clinical tests of body composition (under water weighing, potassium counter, etc) are expensive and time consuming. Simple and reasonably accurate estimates can be made from measures of girth and skinfold thickness.

The following procedures are recommended for assessing body composition from skinfold thickness:

FIGURE 37

STRETCHING EXERCISES BEFORE BEDTIME OR TV

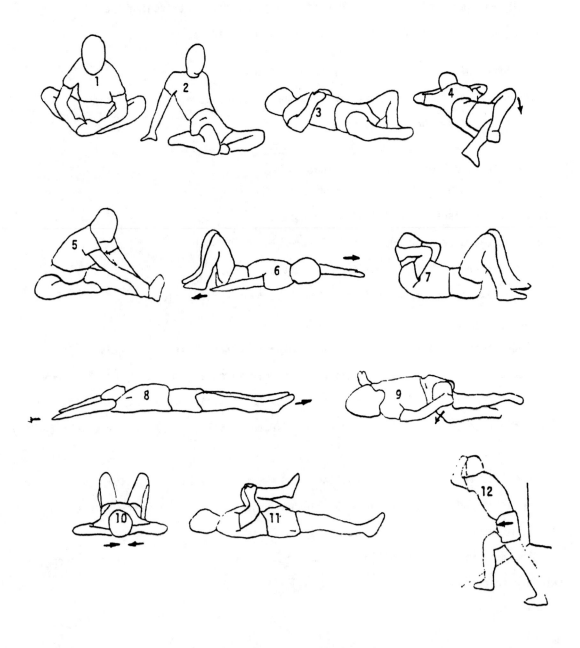

(1) Select skeletal landmarks:

    a) Chest (males) - diagonal fold one-half of the distance between the anterior axillary line and the nipple.

    b) Abdomen (males) - vertical fold adjacent to and approximately 2 centimeters laterally from the umibilicus.

    c) Thigh (males and females) - vertical fold on the anterior thigh midway between the hip and knee joints.

    d) Suprailiac (females) - diagonal fold on the crest of the ilium at the midaxillary line.

    e) Subscapular - fold on diagonal line running from vertebral border one centimeter from the inferior angle of the scapula.

(2) Grasp skinfold at each site firmly between the thumb and index finger.

(3) Place caliper on the site approximately .25 to .50 inch from the thumb and fingers.

(4) Make at least two measurements at each sit, if these differ by more than 1 mm, make a third measurement.

(5) Use the mean of the 2 or 3 trials as the criterion score for each site.

(6) Record Data on appropriate form (Table 43 for males and females).

(7) Convert skinfold sites to predict body density (Table 43).

(8) Compute body density (Table 43).

(9) Convert body density to % fat (Table 44).

(10) Determine classification for body fatness (Table 44).

(11) Calculate fat weight, where FW = (weight X % Fat) ÷ 100.

(12) Calculate lean weight, where LW = body weight - FW

(13) Calculate ideal body weight, where

    a) Males (12% Fat): IDBW = LBW ÷ .88

    b) Females (18% Fat): IDBW - LBW ÷ .82

(14) Determine weight to be lost or gained, where weight loss or gain = Total weight - IDBW.

TABLE 43
RECORD FORMS FOR SKINFOLD DATA

<u>Men</u>

Chest   _____ mm X .000065 = _____

Subscapular   _____ mm X .00055 = _____

Thigh   _____ mm X .00080 = _____

Density = 1.0916 - chest - subscapular - thigh
(gm/cc)

Density = 1.0916 - ____ - ____ - ____ = ____
(gm/cc)

<u>Women</u>

Suprailiac   _____ mm X .0008

Thigh   _____ mm X .0011

Density (gm/cc) = 1.0852 - suprailiac - thigh

Density (gm/cc) = 1.0852 - _____ - _____ = _____

TABLE 44
TABLE TO CONVERT DENSITY TO PERCENT FAT[a]

Density	Percent Fat	Density	Percent Fat	Density	Percent Fat
1.000	45.00	1.033	29.19	1.066	14.35
1.001	44.51	1.034	28.72	1.067	13.92
1.002	44.01	1.035	28.26	1.068	13.48
1.003	43.52	1.036	27.80	1.069	13.05
1.004	43.03	1.037	27.34	1.070	12.62
1.005	42.54	1.038	26.88	1.071	12.18
1.006	42.05	1.039	26.42	1.072	11.75
1.007	41.56	1.040	25.96	1.073	11.32
1.008	41.07	1.041	25.50	1.074	10.89
1.009	40.58	1.042	25.05	1.075	10.47
1.010	40.10	1.043	24.59	1.076	10.04
1.011	39.61	1.044	24.14	1.077	9.51
1.012	39.13	1.045	23.68	1.078	9.18
1.013	38.65	1.046	23.23	1.079	8.76
1.014	38.17	1.047	22.78	1.080	8.33
1.015	37.68	1.048	22.33	1.081	7.91
1.016	37.20	1.049	21.88	1.082	7.49
1.017	36.73	1.050	21.43	1.083	7.06
1.018	36.25	1.051	20.98	1.084	6.64
1.019	35.77	1.052	20.53	1.085	6.22
1.020	35.29	1.053	20.09	1.086	5.80
1.021	34.82	1.054	19.64	1.087	5.38
1.022	34.34	1.055	19.19	1.088	4.96
1.023	33.87	1.056	18.75	1.089	4.55
1.024	33.40	1.057	18.31	1.090	4.13
1.025	32.93	1.058	17.86	1.091	3.71
1.026	32.46	1.059	17.42	1.092	3.30
1.027	31.99	1.060	16.98	1.093	2.88
1.028	31.52	1.061	16.54	1.094	2.47
1.029	31.05	1.062	16.10	1.095	2.05
1.030	30.58	1.063	15.66	1.096	1.64
1.031	30.12	1.064	15.23	1.097	1.23
1.032	29.65	1.065	14.79	1.098	0.82

Density _____ Percent Fat _____

(Sum of conversion)

[a]Siri Percent Fat Formula: % Fat = $\dfrac{4.950}{\text{density}}$ - 4.50 X 100

TABLE 45

ASSESSING BODY BUILD*

Chest. At the nipple line and at the midpoint of a normal breath.
Waist. At the minimal abdominal girth, below the rib cage and just above the top of the hip bone.
Hips. At the level of the symphsis pubis in front, at the maximal protusion of the buttocks in back. Be sure your feet are together when measuring this circumference.
Thigh. At the crotch level and just below the fold of the buttocks (gluteal fold).
Calf. At the maximal circumference.
Ankle. At the minimal circumference, usually just above the ankle bones.
Upper Arm. At the maximal circumference; with arm extended, palm up.
Wrist. At the most minimal circumference; with arm extended, palm up.

    The charts below give recommended girth proportions for women and men. These serve only as a general reference based on measurements of many people who we would classify as trim and well proportioned. Record your measurements. After 8 to 10 weeks of physical fitness conditioning (such as jog-walk-jog, conditioning exercises and maybe modification of your diet), have yourself measured again for changes.

    Recommended girth proportions for women:

Bust should measure same as hips.
Waist should measure 10 inches less than bust or hips.
Hips should measure same as bust.
Thighs should measure 6 inches less than waist.
Calves should measure 6 to 7 inches less than thighs.
Ankles should measure 5 to 6 inches less than calves.
Upper arm should measure twice the size of the wrist.

    Recommended girth proportions for men:

Chest should measure same as hips.
Waist should measure 5 to 7 inches less than chest or hips.
Hips should measure same as chest.
Thighs should measure 8 to 10 inches less than waist.
Calves should measure 7 to 8 inches less than thighs.
Ankles should measure 6 to 7 inches less than calves.
Upper arm should measure twice the size of the wrist.

* Getchell (1979)

If you do not have access to skinfold calipers, physique (body build) can be evaluated from a series of girths. Measurement and calculation procedures for assessing body build are depicted in Table 45.

Day 1

Begin the day by completing the morning stretching exercises as soon after rising as possible (Figure 17). These activities will wake you up and prepare you for the day ahead. Individuals who train first thing in the morning might elect to skip these exercises and do the specific stretching routine recommended to preceed training. If workouts are held later in the day, participants should do the specific stretching warm-up exercises recommended for aerobic training (jogging, cycling, swimming, etc). Following warm-up, complete the aerobic portion of the training program, then cool-down for 5-10 minutes and do the post-training stretching exercises

If strength training is done on the same day as aerobic conditioning, it should be completed following aerobic work. If done on alternate days, strength training should be preceeded by the specific warm-up activities depicted in Figure 30. At various times during the day, especially if you are required to sit, stand or ride for an hour or more, complete the activities in Figure 36. Finally, before retiring for the evening, complete the stretching exercises depicted in Figure 37 and complete the abdominal exercises depicted in Figure 16 and/or Table 32. These exercises will reduce tension and fatigue and enable you to enjoy a more restful sleep.

APPENDIX A
THE FAST FOOD CALORIE COUNTER

The figures listed below indicate the caloric value of specific fast foods. Also listed are the minutes that you would have to run in order to work-off the calories consumed. These figures are computed for individuals who weigh 120, 170 or 200 pounds and are based on a running speed of 201 meters per minute (8:00 min mile pace). Individuals who run at a slower pace must run longer; e.g., a 120 pounder who eats a Burger King Cheeseburger (305 cal.) must run for 25 minutes if he runs at 8:00 min/mile pace and 31 minutes if he runs at 10:00 min/mile pace. Individuals who run slower than an 8:00 min/mile pace should add approximately 3 minutes of running for each minute over 8 minutes that it takes to run a mile.

| | CAL. | Running Time (min) | | |
		120 lb	170 lb	200 lb
BURGER KING				
Cheeseburger	365	25	18	15
French Fries	220	18	13	11
Hamburger	230	19	14	11
Hamburger, Double	325	27	19	16
Shake, Chocolate	361	30	21	18
Whopper	630	53	37	32
Whopper Junior	285	25	17	14
COLONEL SANDERS'				
KENTUCKY FRIED CHICKEN				
Dinner (Fried Chicken, Mashed potatoes, Coleslaw, Rolls);				
2-Piece Dinner--Original	595	50	35	30
Crispy	665	55	39	33
3-Piece Dinner -Original	980	82	58	49
Crispy	1,170	89	63	54
DAIRY QUEEN/BRAZIER				
"Bosn's Mate" Fish Sandwich	340	28	20	17
"Brazier"	250	21	15	13
"Brazier" Barbecue	280	23	16	14
"Brazier" Cheeseburger	310	26	18	16
"Brazier" Chili Dog	530	28	19	17
"Brazier" Dog	270	23	16	14
"Brazier" French Fries	200	19	12	10
"Brazier" Onion Rings	300	25	18	16
Big "Brazier"	510	43	30	26
Big "Brazier" Cheeseburger	600	50	35	30
Big "Brazier" Deluxe	540	45	32	27
Super "Brazier" Chili Dog	570	48	34	28
Super "Brazier" Dog	300	25	18	15
Super "Brazier"/The "Half- Pounder"	850	71	52	43
Ice Creams				
Banana Splits	580	44	11	27
Buster Bar	390	33	23	20
Dairy Queen Cones				
Small	110	9	7	5
Medium	230	19	14	12
Large	340	28	20	17
Dairy Queen Dipped Cones				
Small	160	13	9	
Medium	310	26	18	11
Large	450	38	26	23
Dairy Queen Malts				
Small	400	33	24	20
Medium	580	48	34	28
Large	830	69	49	42

| | CAL. | Running Time (min) | | |
		120 lb	170 lb	200 lb
Dairy Queen Sundaes				
Small	190	16	11	9
Medium	300	25	18	15
Large	430	36	25	22
Dilly Bar	240	20	14	12
DQ Sandwich	190	16	11	10
Hot Fudge "Brownie Delight Sundae"	580	48	34	29
Parfait	400	38	27	23
ARTHUR TREACHER'S				
Chips (per serving)	274	23	16	14
Coleslaw	122	10	7	6
Fish (2 pieces)	344	29	20	17
BASKIN-ROBBINS				
One Scoop				
Ice Creams, all flavors	between 133 and 148	12	8	7
Sherberts and Ices	139	12	8	7
BURGER CHEF				
Big Chef	333	28	20	17
French Fries	240	20	14	12
Hamburger	230	21	15	13
Shake, Chocolate	310	26	18	16
Super Chef	530	44	31	27
DUNKIN DONUTS				
Donuts (including rings, sticks, crullers)	240	20	14	12
Donuts, yeast-raised (add 5-10 calories for glaze	160	13	9	8
Fancies (includes coffee rolls, Danish, etc)	215	18	13	11
Munchkins, yeast-raised	26	2	2	1
Cake, including chocolate cake	240	20	14	12
GINO'S				
Apple Pie	198	17	12	10
Cheeseburger	336	28	20	17
Coke (regular)	117	10	7	6
Coke (giant)	181	15	11	9
Dinner Roll	51	4	3	3
Fry (regular)	195	16	11	10
Fry (giant)	274	23	16	14
Hamburger	289	24	17	14
Fried Chicken (1 piece)	290	24	17	15
Orange (regular)	140	12	8	7
Orange (giant)	217	18	13	11
RootBeer (regular)	128	16	8	6

| | CAL. | Running Time (min) | | |
		120 lb	170 lb	200 lb
GINO'S (cont'd)				
Shake, Vanilla (regular)	338	28	20	17
Shake, Vanilla (giant)	524	44	31	26
Sirloiner	514	43	30	26
Sirloiner (Cheese)	609	51	36	31
LONG JOHN SILVER'S				
Fish & Chips, Clowslaw				
2-piece Dinner	955	83	59	50
3-piece Dinner	1,190	99	70	60
MCDONALD'S				
Apple Pie	265	22	16	13
Big Mac	557	46	33	28
Cheeseburger	309	26	18	15
Egg McMuffin	312	26	18	10
Fillet-O-Fish	406	34	24	20
French Fries	215	18	13	11
Hamburger	249	21	15	12
Hamburger, Double	330	28	19	17
Hot Cakes with Butter	272	23	16	14
Muffin	136	11	8	7
Pork Sausage	235	20	14	12
1/4 Pounder	414	35	24	21
1/4 Pounder with Cheese	521	43	31	26
Scrambles Eggs	175	15	10	9
Shake, Chocolate	317	24	19	16
Shake, Strawberry	315	24	19	16
Shake, Vanilla	322	28	19	17
PIZZA HUT				
1/2 of 13-inch Cheese Pizza				
Thick Crust	900	75	53	45
Thin Crust	850	71	50	43
1/2 of 15-inch Cheese Pizza				
Thick Crust	1,200	100	71	60
Thin Crust	1,130	96	68	58
1/2 of 10-inch Pizza (Thin Crust)				
Beef	488	41	29	24
Cheese	436	36	26	22
Pepperoni	459	38	27	23
Pork	466	39	27	23
Supreme	475	40	28	24
15-inch Pepperoni Pizza (Thin Crust)	1,377	114	81	69

	CAL.	Running Time (min)		
		120 lb	170 lb	200 lb
RUSTLER STEAK HOUSE				
Baked Potato	251	19	14	12
Dressing (Blue Cheese)	151	13	9	8
Dressing (French)	122	10	7	6
Dressing (Italian)	166	14	10	8
Dressing (Thousand Island)	150	13	9	7
Jello-Cherry	250	6	4	4
Pickle	2	2	1	1
Potato Chips	82	7	5	4
Pudding, Chocolate	144	12	9	7
Roll (Butter)	40	3	2	1
Roll (Rustler)	120	10	7	6
Roll (Twisted)	182	7	5	4
Rib Eye	369	31	22	19
Rustler's (Strip)	1,086	91	64	54
Salad	13	1	8	6
Steak (Chopped) 4 oz.	327	27	19	16
Steak (Chopped) 8 oz.	653	54	38	33
T-Bone	1,532	128	90	77
TACO-BELL				
Beans (Whipped) Burito	345	29	20	17
Bell Burger	243	20	14	12
Enchirito	391	33	23	20
Frijoles	231	19	14	12
Taco	146	12	9	7
Tostado	206	17	12	10
WHITE CASTLE				
Cheeseburger	198	17	12	10
Fish Sandwich	200	17	12	10
French Fries	219	18	13	11
Hamburger	165	14	10	8
Milk Shake	213	18	13	11
Onion Rings	341	28	20	17

APPENDIX B
STRENGTH TRAINING PROCEDURES
FREE WEIGHTS

1. Modified Clean and Power Press

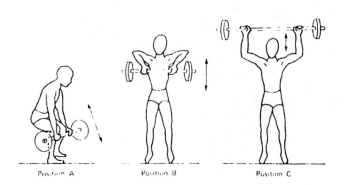

Position A   Position B   Position C

From the crouch position, using an overhand grip, lift the bar with a very fast pull from the floor, employing the legs and hips until the legs are straight. At this point the bar should have acquired momentum. As the body straightens, the upward pull of the bar is continued by rising on the toes and pulling with the arms, keeping the bar close to the legs and body. When the bar reaches shoulder level the player dips under it with all of the speed possible to a half-squat. This action momentarily takes the weight off the wrists, enabling him to turn the wrists under and get his chest beneath the bar. It is important that the wrist and elbows be thrust under rapidly in order to better support the bar as it is brought to the chest and shoulders. The bar should travel from the floor to shoulder level in one continuous movement. Thrust the weight from the chest to an overhead position by straightening the legs and extending the arms. Return to the starting position and repeat. Use heavier weights than in the overhead press exercise and execute the thrusting movement with as much arm, shoulder and leg force as can be brought into play.

2. Squats

Start with relatively light weights during
the learning stages. The bar should
rest across the shoulders and back
of the neck with the hands grasping it
at somewhat greater than shoulder-
width apart. The exerciser puts the
bar in position by executing a clean and
press and lowering the bar to the shoulders
behind the neck. When very heavy
weights are desired it becomes necessary
to have two assistants place the bar
across the shoulders. The feet should
be comfortably positioned, usually about
shoulder-width apart with the heels
elevated and a two-inch board. With
the back kept straight and the chest
high the body is lowered into a three-
quarter squat position and raised to
a starting position as many times as
desired, inhaling as the legs flex and
exhaling while they extend. Beginners
need to be cautioned against bending at
the waist. A pad may be placed under
the bar at the neck. The squat
exercise is probably best for development of powerful legs and hips. If
there is difficulty stopping at the 3/4
squat position, a good precaution is to
place a low bench behind the legs so
that the trainee will sit on the bench
rather than continue to the full squat
position. The bench would be 1-2 inches
lower than the knees.

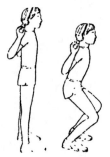

AS YOU SQUAT:

1. BACK STRAIGHT
2. HEAD UP AND EYES AHEAD
3. LET THE TAIL GO DOWN FIRST
4. KEEP FEET FLAT OR HEELS ON A 2-INCH BOARD
5. DO NOT PERMIT THE KNEES TO MOVE IN TOWARD EACH OTHER
6. DO NOT COME TO A COMPLETE STOP-MERELY TOUCH-THEN STAND

3. Bench Press

Assume a supine position on the bench with
the head, shoulders and hips contacting it
and the legs straddling it, feet flat on the
floor. Take the barbell off the rack or
from two assistants in a straight-arm
supporting position. Use an overhand grip
and grasp the barbell slightly wider than
shoulder-width. Lower the bar to the chest
and press it to the straight-arm position.
Refrain from bringing the buttocks off
the bench during the press. Inhale while
pressing and exhale as the arms are locked.
Holding the elbows wide will bring the
chest muscles into greater use.

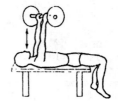

4. Toe Raises

Place the barbell across the back of the
neck and shoulders, hands grasping the
bar at slightly more than shoulder-width.
Place the toes on a 2-3 inch board and
raise forcefully to full height on the
toes. Lower to original position and
repeat. Position the feet so the toes
point out, in and straight ahead to
vary the exercise.

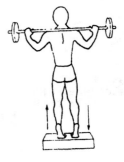

5. Triceps Press

Using an overhand grip, grasp the bar
with the hands spaced no more than 10
inches apart. Clean and press the bar,
positioning it across the back of the
neck, and shoulders. The elbows should
point directly up. From this position
press the bar to a full overhead extension and return to the starting
position. Keep the head bent slightly
forward to avoid contacting the bar.

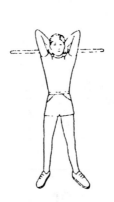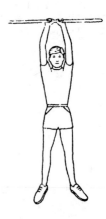

6. Curls

Using the underhand grip, grasp the bar with
the hands shoulder-width apart. Stand
erect, the bar hanging at a thigh rest
position. The feet should be comfortably
spread. Keeping the upper arms motionless
and close to the body, flex the arms at
the elbow joint until the bar touches the
chest. Return the bar in the same arc.

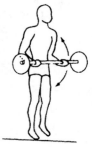

7. Straight-Arm Pullover

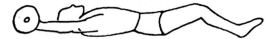

Lie supine on the floor or bench and hold the barbell at full arm extension over the chest. The overhand grip is used and the hands are spaced slightly wider than shoulder width. Keeping the arms straight, lower the bar in an arch to a position directly above the head and, after a brief pause, return it in the same manner. Inhale deeply during the first movement and exhale as the bar is returned.

8. Lateral Dumbell Raises

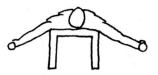

While supine on an exercise bench, hold a pair of dumbells directly over the chest with palms facing in. Bend the arms slightly and keep them bent throughout the exercise. Lower the weights in an arc to the sides and return in the same arc to the starting position. Inhale deeply during the first movement and exhale during the second.

APPENDIX C
STRENGTH TRAINING PROCEDURES
UNIVERSAL GYM

* Denotes starting weight.

1. Bench Press   *100 lbs

Lie on back on bench. Grasp
bar in hands with hands slightly
wider than shoulders. Press to
straight-arm position and slowly
lower.

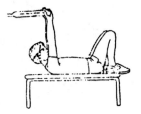

2. Lateral Pulls   *80-90 lbs

Squat

Kneel down. Grasp bar at ends.
Pull bar down until it touches
the bump on back of the neck.
Slowly return and then pull-down
to mid-chest level in front of body.
Alternate pulls behind and in front
of body.

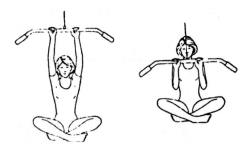

3. Leg Press & Calf Extension

Sit in chair. Place feet on bottom
supports. Extend hips and legs.
*180 lbs
Calf Ext. Extend legs and then
extend toes. Repeat sets with toes
together-heels apart and with heels
together-toes apart. *180 lbs

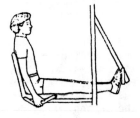

4. Biceps Curl   *30-40 lbs

Grasp bar in hands. Pull (curl)
bar to chest. Return slowly.

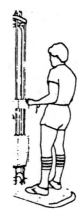

5. Leg Extension   *40-50 lbs

Sit on bench. Place ankles
behind pads. Extend knees
completely and HOLD for 2-seconds.
Slowly lower.

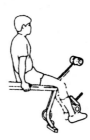

6. Leg Curl   *20-30 lbs

Lie on bench on stomach. Place
heels under pads. Curl heels to
buttocks. HOLD for 2-seconds.

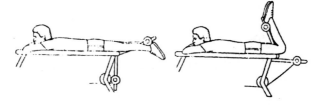

7. Triceps Press   *30-40 lbs

Stand erect. Grasp bar used in
Lateral Pulls in the center with
hands together, palms down and
elbows almost together. Extend
elbows completely until hands
are at waist level. Return slowly.

8. Pull Overs   *30-40 lbs

Lie on back at Station No. 4,
Biceps Curl, with head towards
machine. Grasp bar with palms
up and arm straight. Pull bar
in an arc (circle) over head to
waist level. Return slowly.

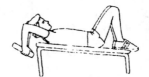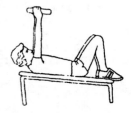

NAUTILUS TRAINING PRINCIPLES

General procedures To be followed on all machines where the regular (positive- negative) form of exercise is performed:

1. On any machine where seat adjustments or body positioning can be varied, make certain that the rotational axis of the cam is directly parallel to the rotational axis (joint) of the body part that is being moved.

2. Position your body in a straightly aligned manner. Avoid twisting or shifting your weight during the movement.

3. Never squeeze hand grips tightly, but maintain a loose comfortable grip (a tight grip elevates blood pressure).

4. Lift the resistance (positive work) to the count of two . . . pause . . . lower the resistance (negative work) slowly and smoothly while counting to four.

5. For full-range strength and flexibility (and protection against injury) your range of movement on each machine should be as great as possible.

6. Breathe normally. Try not to hold your breath while straining.

7. Perform each exercise for 8 to 12 repetitions.

    a. Begin with a weight you can comfortably do 8 times.

    b. Stay with that weight until you can perform 12 strict repetitions. On the following workout, increase the weight (approximately 5%) and go back to 8 repetitions.

    c. Ideally, on every workout you should progress in repetitions and/or resistance.

8. For best cardiorespiratory (heart - lungs) conditioning, move quickly from machine to machine (this speed does not apply to the actual exercises). The longer the rest between machines, the less effective the cardiorespiratory conditioning.

9. When possible, follow your routine as the exercises are numbered on your workout sheet; however any time the machine you are to do next is being used, go to another exercise and then return to the machine that was in use.

10. All compound and double machines were designed to make use of the pre exhaustion principle (where a single joint exercise is used to pre-exhaust a given muscle and a multiple joint exercise is used to force the exhausted muscle to work even harder); therefore, it is important to move very quickly (in less than 3 seconds) from the primary exercise to the secondary exercise.

11. Your training session should include a maximum of 12 exercises. 4 to 6 for the lower body and 6 to 8 for the upper body a compound machine counts as two exercises).

12. Exercise the larger muscle groups first and proceed down to the smaller muscle groups (hips, thighs, back, shoulders, chest, arms, and neck).

13. Your entire workout should take from 20 to 30 minutes.

14. The time lapse between exercise sessions should be at least 48 hours and not more than 96 hours.

DUOsymmetric/
POLYcontractile
HIP AND BACK MACHINE

(Buttocks and lower back)

1. Enter machine from front by separating movement arms.
2. Lay on back with both legs over roller pads.
3. Align hip joints with axes of cams.
4. Fasten seat belt and grasp handles lightly.
5. Seat belt should be snug, but not too tight, as back must be arched at completion of movement.
6. From bent-legged position, extend both legs and at same time push back with hands.
7. Holding one leg at full extension, allow other leg to bend and come back as far as possible.
8. Stretch.
9. Push out until it joins other leg at extension.
10. Pause, arch lower back, and contract buttocks.
11. Repeat with other leg.

Important: In contracted position, keep legs straight, knees together, and toes pointed.

POLY-CONTRACTILE HIP AND BACK MACHINE

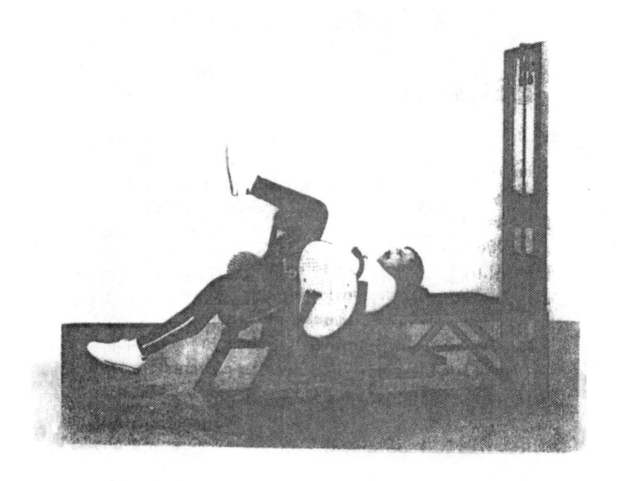

LEG CURL MACHINE

(Hamstrings)
1. Lay face down on machine.
2. Place feet under roller pads with knees just over edge of bench.
3. Lightly grasp handles to keep body from moving.
4. Curl legs and try to touch heels to buttocks.
5. When lower legs are pertpendicular to bench, lift buttocks to increase movement.
6. Pause at point of full muscular contraction.
7. Slowly lower resistance and repeat.

Important: Top of foot should be flexed toward knee throughout movement.

LEG CURL MACHINE

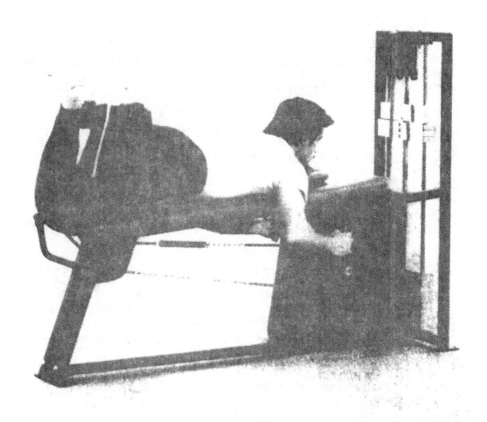

COMPOUND LEG MACHINE

Leg Extension (Frontal thighs or quadriceps)

1. In a seated position, place feet behind roller pads with knees snug against seat.
2. Adjust seat back to comfortable position.
3. Keep head and shoulders against seat back.
4. Straighten both legs smoothly.
5. Pause.
6. Slowly lower resistance and repeat.
7. After final repetition, immediately do leg press.

Leg Press (Quadriceps, hamstrings, and buttocks)

1. Sit erect and pull seat back forward.
2. Flip down foot pads.
3. Place both feet on pads with toes pointed slightly inward.
4. Straighten both legs in a controlled manner.
5. Return to stretched position and repeat.

Important: Avoid tightly gripping handles and do not grit teeth or tense neck or face muscles during either movement.

COMPOUND LEG MACHINE

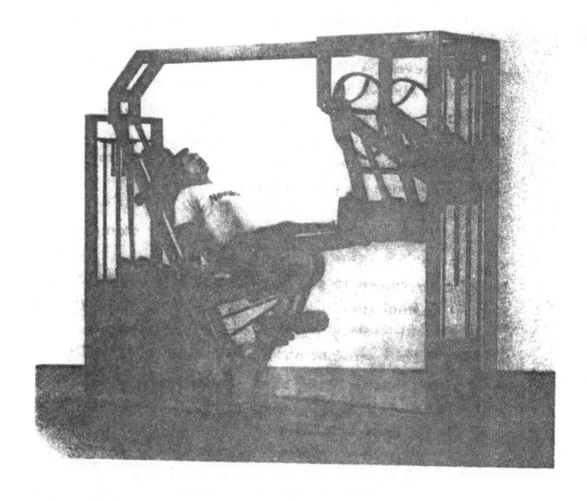

PULLOVER / TORSO ARM MACHINE

Pullover (Latissimus dorsi muscles of the back and other torso muscles)

1. Adjust seat so shoulder joints are in line with axes of cams.
2. Assume erect position and fasten seat belt tightly.
3. Leg press foot pedal until elbow pads are about chin level.
4. Place elbows on pads.
5. Hands should be open and resting on curved portion of bar.
6. Remove legs from pedal and slowly rotate elbows as far back as possible.
7. Stretch.
8. Rotate elbows down until bar touches stomach.
9. Pause.
10. Slowly return to stretched position and repeat.
11. After final repetition, immediately do pulldown.

Important: Look straight ahead during movement. Do not move head or torso. Do not grip tightly with hands.

Torso Arm Pulldown (Latissimus dorsi of back and biceps of upper arms)

1. Lower seat to bottom for maximum stretch.
2. Grasp overhead bar with palms-up grip.
3. Keep head and shoulders against seat back.
4. Pull bar to chest.
5. Pause.
6. Slowly return to stretched position and repeat.

PULLOVER/TORSO ARM MACHINE

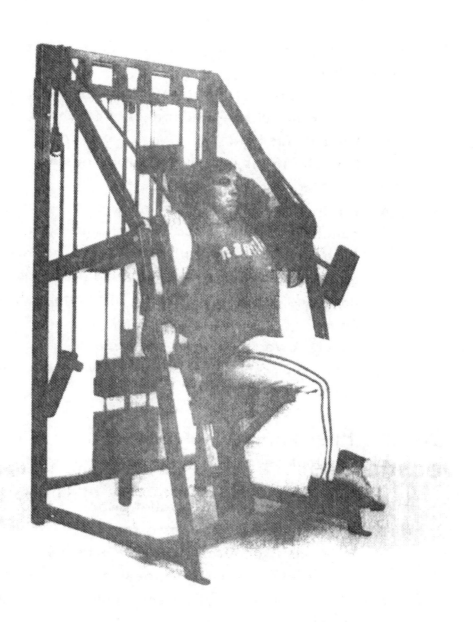

DOUBLE CHEST MACHINE

Arm Cross (Pectoralis majors of the chest and deltoids of shoulders)

1. Adjust seat until shoulders (when elbows are together) are directly under axes of overhead cams.
2. Fasten seat belt.
3. Place forearms behind and firmly against movement arm pads.
4. Lightly grasp handles (thumb should be around handle) and keep head against seat back.
5. Push with forearms and try to touch elbows together in front of chest. (Movement can also be done one arm at a time in an alternate fashion.)
6. Pause.
7. Slowly lower resistance and repeat.
8. After final repetition, immediately do decline press.

Decline Press (Chest, shoulders, and triceps of arms)

1. Use foot pedal to raise handles into starting position.
2. Grasp handles with parallel grip.
3. Keep head back and torso erect.
4. Press bars forward in controlled fashion.
5. Slowly lower resistance keeping elbows wide.
6. Stretch at point of full extension and repeat pressing movement.

DOUBLE CHEST MACHINE

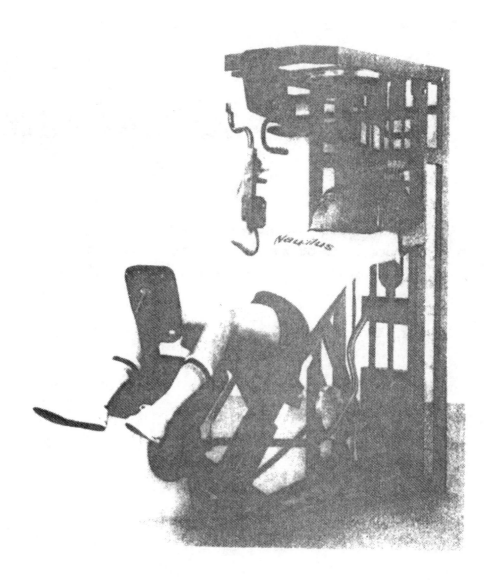

ROWING TORSO MACHINE

(Deltoids and trapezius)

1. Sit with back toward weight stack.
2. Place arms between pads and cross arms.
3. Bend arms in rowing fashion as far back as possible.
4. Pause.
5. Slowly return to starting position and repeat.

Important: Keep arms parallel to floor at all times.

ROWING TORSO MACHINE

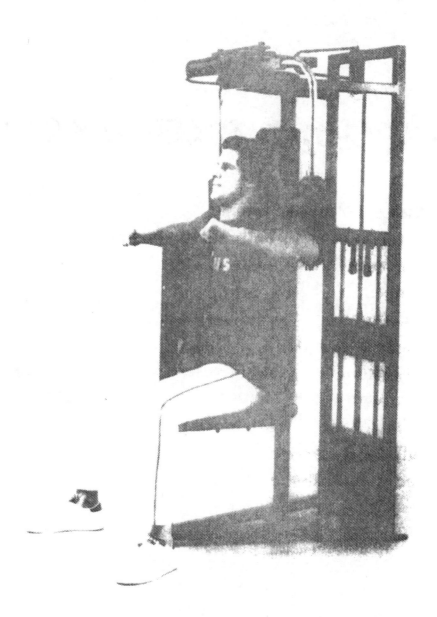

COMPOUND BICEP MACHINE

(Biceps of the upper arms)
1. Adjust seat so both elbows are in line with axes of cams.
2. Place thighs on seat.
3. Arms should be fully extended as hand grips are lightly grasped.
4. Curl one arm behind neck.
5. Pause.
6. Slowly lower resistance.
7. Repeat with other arm.

COMPOUND BICEP MACHINE

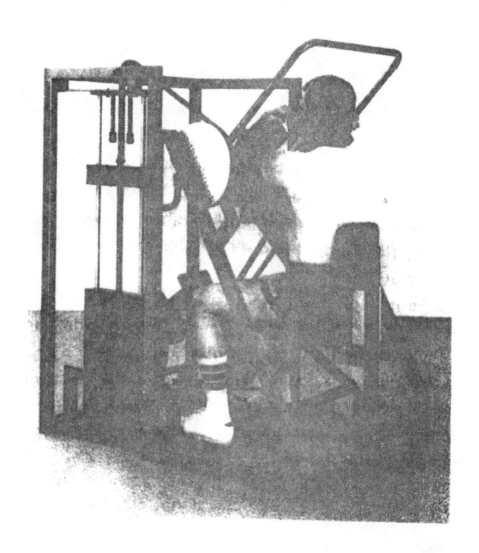

COMPOUND TRICEP MACHINE

(Triceps of upper arms)
1. Adjust seat so elbows are in line with axis of cam.
2. Keep elbows against pads, head and shoulders against seat back, and thighs on seat.
3. Lightly grasp handles with palms on pads.
4. Smoothly extend arms.
5. Pause.
6. Slowly return to stretched position and repeat.

Important: For proper performance elbows must be held against pads at all times.

COMPOUND TRICEP MACHINE

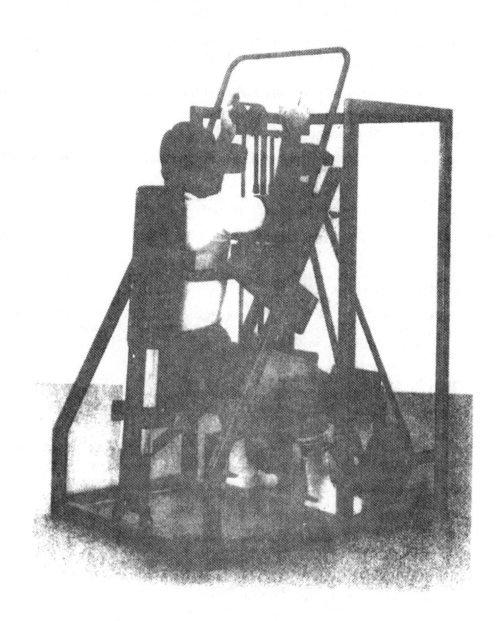

REFERENCES

1. Adams, W. C. "Influence of age, sex and body weight on energy expenditure of bicycle riding." Journal of Applied Physiology. 22:538-545, 1975.

2. Allen, T., F. Byrd and D. Smith. "Hemodynamic consequences of circuit weight training." Research Quarterly, 47:299-306, 1976.

3. American College of Sports Medicine. "Position statement on prevention of heat injuries during distance running." Medicine and Science in Sports. 7:vii-ix, 1975.

4. American Heart Association. Heart Facts-1979. American Heart Association, Dallas, Texas, 1978.

5. Anderson, B. Stretching. Bolinas, Ca: Shelter Publications, 1980.

6. Anderson, B. "The 1979 runner's world shoe survey." Runner's World. 13:62-107, 1979.

7. Asmussen, E. "Observations on experimental muscular soreness." Acta Rheumatologica Scandinavica. 2:109-116, 1956.

8. Astrand, I. "Aerobic work capacity in men and women." Acta Physiologica Scandinavica. (supplement) 49:169, 1960.

9. Astrand, P. O. and K. Rodahl. Textbook of Work Physiology. New York: McGraw Hill Book Company, 1970.

10. Baldwin, K. M., J. S. Reitman, R. L. Terjung, W. W. Winder and J. O. Holloszy. "Respiratory capacity of white, red and intermediate muscle: adaptive responses to exercise." American Journal of Physiology. 222:373-378, 1972.

11. Balke, B. "A simple field test for the assessment of physical fitness." CARI Report 63-6. Civil Aeromedical Research Institute Federal Aviation Agency, Oklahoma City, 1963.

12. Balke, B. and R. Clark. "Cardiopulmonary and metabolic effects of physical training." Health and Fitness in the Modern World. A. Larson (ed). Chicago: The Athletic Institute. 1961.

13. Barry, A. "The effects of physical conditioning on older individuals. Work capacity, circulatory-respiratory function, and work electrocardiogram." Journal of Gerontology. 21:182, 1966.

14. Bassler, T. J. "Marathon running and immunity to heart disease." Physician and Sports Medicine, 3(4):77-80, 1975.

15. Becklace, M. "Influence of age and sex on exercise cardiac output." Journal of Applied Physiology. 20:938, 1965.

16. Behnke, A. R. and J. H. Wilmore. Evaluation and Regulation of Body Build and Composition. Englewood Cliffs, N. J: Prentice-Hall, 1974

17. Beischer, D. E. and A. R. Fregly. *Animals and Man in Space, A Chronology and Annotated Bibliography Through the Year 1960*. ONR Rep. ACR-64 (USMAM Monograph 5), Department of the Navy, 1961.

18. Benestae. A. "Trainability of older men." *Acta. Med. Scand.* 178:321, 1965.

19. Berger, R. A. "Effect of varied weight training programs on strength." *Research Quarterly*. 33:168-181, 1962.

20. Berger, R. A. "Optimum repetitions for the development of strength." *Research Quarterly*. 33:334-338, 1962.

21. Booth, F. W. and C. M. Tipton. "Ligamentous strength measurements in pre-pubescent and pubescent rats." *Growth*. 34:177-185, 1970.

22. Bray, G. "Effect of caloric restriction on energy expenditure in obese subjects." *Lancet*. 2:397-398, 1969.

23. Brynteson, P. H. "The effects of training frequencies of the retention of cardiovascular fitness." Unpublished Doctoral Dissertation, Springfield College, 1969.

24. Campbell, D. E. "Heart rates of selected male college freshmen during a season of basketball." *Research Quarterly*. 39:880-887, 1968.

25. Campbell, D. E. "Maintenance of strength during a season of sports partici-pation." *American Corrective Therapy Journal*. 21:193-195, 1967.

26. Clauser, C. E. *Weight, Volume and Center of Mass of Segments of the Human Body*. NASA. AMRL-TR-69-70, 1969.

27. Coleman, A. E. and P. Kreuzer. "Aerobic and anaerobic responses to a season of college basketball." *Journal of Sports Medicine and Physical Fitness*. 14:26-30, 1974.

28. Coleman, A. E. "Aerobic capacity of professional baseball players." Unpublished data, 1978.

29. Coleman, A. E. "Body composition of major league baseball players," Unpublished data, 1978.

30. Coleman, A. E. "Comparison of isometric and isotonic contractions performed on contralateral limbs." *Corrective Therapy*. 23:163-166, 1969.

31. Coleman, A. E. "Strength maintenance in athletics: a review." *Montana AAHPER Journal*. 2:28-29, 1970.

32. Coleman, A. E. "Strength maintenance in professional baseball players." Unpublished data, 1978.

33. Coleman, A. E. "Nautilus vs univerals gym training in young women." *Australian Journal of Sports Medicine*. 9:4-7, 1977.

34. Coleman, A. E. "Strength maintenance of college football players." *Kentucky AAHPER Journal*. 6:10-11, 1970.

35. Consolazio, D., R. Johnson and L. Pecora. *Physiological Measurements of Metabolic Methods in Man.* New York: McGraw-Hill Book Company, Inc., 1963

36. Cooper, K. H. *Aerobics.* New York: Bantam Books, 1968.

37. Cooper, K. H. "Correlation between field and treadmill testing as a means of assessing maximal oxygen intake." *Journal of the American Medical Association.* 203:201-204, 1968.

38. Cooper, K. H. "Guidelines in the management of the exercising patient." *Journal of the American Medical Association.* 211:1663-1667, 1970.

39. Cooper, K. H., M. L. Pollock, R. P. Martin, S. R. White, A. C. Linerud and A. Jackson, "Physical fitness levels vs selected coronary risk factors." *Journal of the American Medical Association.* 236(2):166-169, 1976.

40. Cooper, K. H. Personal communication, 1980.

41. Cooper, K. H. *The Aerobics Way.* New York: Bantam Books, 1977.

42. Cooper, K. H. *The Aerobics Way.* New York, Bantam Books, 1978.

43. Cooper, K. H. *The New Aerobics.* New York: J. B. Lippincott, 1970.

44. Costill, D. L., J. Daniels, W. Evans, W. Fink, G. Krahenbuhl and B. Saltin. "Skeletal muscle enzymes and fiber composition in male and female track athletes." *Journal of Applied Physiology.* 40:149-154, 1976.

45. Costill, D. L. Personal communication. October, 1979.

46. Costill, D. L. "The drinking runner." *The Complete Diet Guide for Runners and Other Athletes.* Higdon, H. (ed.). Mountain View, Ca: World Publications, 1978.

47. Costill, D. L., W. J. Fink and M. L. Pollock, "Muscle fiber composition and enzyme activities of elite distance runners." *Medicine and Science in Sports.* 8:96-100, 1976.

48. Cotton, D. "Relationship of the duration of sustained voluntary isometric contractions to changes in endurance and strength." *Research Quarterly.* 38:366-374, 1967.

49. Cureton, T. K. "A physical fitness case study of joie ray (improving physical fitness from 60 to 70 years of age)." *Journal of the Association for Physical and Mental Rehabilitation.* 18:64, 1964.

50. Cureton, T. K. and E. F. Phillips, "Physical fitness changes in middle-aged men attributable to equal eight week periods of training, non-smoking, and re-training." *Journal of Sports Medicine.* 4:87-93, 1964.

51. Daniels, J. T. Personal communication, 1975.

52. Daniels, J. T., R. Fitts and G. Sheehan. *Conditioning for Distance Running: The Scientific Aspects.* New York: John Wiley, and Sons, 1978.

53. Darden, E. Strength Training Principles: How to Get the Most Out of Your Workouts. Winter Park, Fla: Anna Publishing, Inc., 1977.

54. DeLorme, T. L. and A. L. Watkins, "Techniques of progressive resistance exercise." Archives of Physical and Medical Rehabilitation. 29:263-277, 1948.

55. DeLorme, T. L. "Restoration of muscle power by heavy-resistive exercises." Journal of Bone and Joint Surgery. 27:645-667, 1945.

56. Dempster, W. T. Space Requirements of the Seated Operator.

57. deVries, H. A. Physiology of Exercise for Physical Education and Athletics, 2nd ed. Dubuque, Iowa, W. C. Brown, 1974.

58. Dills, B. D. "Marathoner de mar: physiological studies." Journal of the National Cancer Institute. 35:185, 1965.

59. Drinkwater, B. L. and S. M. Horvath, "Detraining effects on young women," Medicine and Science in Sports. 4:91-95, 1972.

60. Drinkwater, B. L., personal correspondence, 1977.

61. Drinkwater, B. L. "Physiological responses of women to exercise." Exercise and Sport Sciences Reviews. Vol. 1, edited by J. H. Wilmore, New York: Academic Press, 1973.

62. Dubowitz, V. and M. H. Brooks, Muscle Biopsy: A Modern Approach. (Volume II). London: W. B. Saunders Company Ltd., 1973.

63. Edington, D. W. and V. R. Edgerton. The Biology of Physical Activity. Boston: Houghton Mifflin Company, 1976.

64. Ekblom, B., P. O. Astrand, B. Saltin, J. Stenberg and P. Wallstrom. "Effect of training on circulatory response to exercise." Journal of Applied Physiology. 24:518, 1968.

65. Fardy, P. S. "Effects of soccer training and detraining upon selected cardiac and metabolic measures." Research Quarterly, 40:502-508, 1969.

66. Faulkner, J. H. "Physiology of swimming," Research Quarterly. 37:41-54, 1966.

67. Faulkner, J. H. "Pulse rate after 50-meter swims." Research Quarterly, 37: 282-284, 1966.

68. Faulkner, J. A. "The physiology of swimming and diving." Exercise Physiology. Falls, H. B. (ed). New York: Academic Press. 1968.

69. Foster, C. "Physiological requirements of aerobic dancing." Research Quarterly 46:120, 1975.

70. Fox, E. L., Sports Physiology, Philadelphia, PA: W. B. Saunders Company, 1979.

71. Fox, S. M., III. and W. L. Haskell. "Physical activity and the prevention of coronary heart disease." Bullentin of the New York Academy of Medicine, 44:950-967, 1963.

72. Garfield, D. S. "Flexibility and physical performance." InBurk, E. J. (ed). Toward an Understanding of Human Performance. Ithaca, N.Y: Movement Publications, 1977.

73. Gettman. L. R., J. J. Ayres, M. L. Pollock and A. S. Jackson. "The effect of circuit training on strength, cardiorespiratory function and body composition." Medicine and Science in Sports. 10:171-176, 1978.

74. Gettman, L. R., L. A. Culter and T. A. Stratham. "Physiologic changes after 20 weeks of isotonic vs isokinetic circuit weight training." Personal communication, 1979.

75. Gettman, L. R., M. L. Pollock, J. L. Durstine, A. Ward, J. Ayres and A. C. Linnerud. "Physiological responses of men to 1, 3 and 5 days per week training programs." Research Quarterly, 47:638-646, 1976.

76. Gisolfi, C. V. and J. R. Copping, "Thermal effects of prolonged treadmill exercise in the heat." Medicine and Science in Sports. 6:108-113, 1974.

77. Glucksman, M. L. and J. Hirsch. "The response of obese patients to weight reduction." Psychosomatic Medicine. 30:1-11, 1968.

78. Gollnick, P. D., R. B. Armstrong, B. Saltin, C. W. Subert IV, W. L. Sembrowich and R. E. Shepard. "Effect of training on enzyme activity and fiber composition of human skeletal muscle." Journal of Applied Physiology. 34:107-111, 1973.

79. Gollnick, P. D., R. B. Armstrong, C. W. Saubert IV, K. Piehl and B. Saltin. "Enzyme activity and fiber composition in skeletal muscle or untrained and trained men." Journal of Applied Physiology, 33:312-319, 1972.

80. Guess, L. E. "A comparison of two training programs for maintaining increased muscular strength developed during an off-season conditioning program." Unpublished Master of Education Thesis, The University of Texas. Austin, 1967.

81. Guidelines for Graded Exercise Testing and Exercise Prescription. Philadelphia, Lea and Febiger, 1975.

82. Harris, R. "Factors affecting the drop-out rate among members of the Aerobic Activity Center." Personal communication. 1978.

83. Hermansen, L. "Anaerobic energy release." Medicine and Science in Sports, 1:32-38, 1969.

84. Hettinger, T. Physiology of Strength. Springfield, Ill: Charles C. Thomas Publisher, 1961.

85. Higdon, H. Beginner's Running Guide. Mountain View, CA: World Publications, 1973.

86. Hogdon, H. Fitness After Forty. Mountain View, CA: World Publications. 1977.

87. Hockey, R. V. Physical Fitness, The Pathway to Healthful Living. St. Louis, The C. V. Mosby Company, 1973.

88. Hoffmann, L. The Great American Nutrition Hassle. Palo Alto: Mayfield Publishing Company, 1978.

89. Hollmann, W. "Korperliches training als prevention von herz-Kreislanfkran-kneiten. "Hippokrates-Verlag. Stuttgart: 1965.

90. Hultman, E. "Studies on muscle metabolism of glycogen and active phosphate in man with special reference to exercise and diet." Scandinavica Journal of Clinical Laboratory Investigation (Supplement 94), 19:1-63, 1967.

91. Johns, R. J. and V. Wright, "Relative importance of various tissues in joint stiffness." Journal of Applied Physiology. 17:824-828, 1962.

92. Johnson, B. E., J. W. Adamezyk, K. O. Tennoe and S. B. Stromme. "A comparison of concentric and eccentric muscle training." Medicine and Science in Sports. 8:35-38, 1976.

93. Johnson, P. B. et al, Physical Education - A Problem Solving Approach to Health and Fitness. New York: Hold, Rinehart and Winson, 1966.

94. Johnson, R. S. and L. R. Dietlein, Biomedical Results from Skylab. NASA SP-377, 1977.

95. Johnson, R. S., L. F. Dietlein and C. A. Berry. Biomedical Results of Apollo. NASA SP-368, 1975.

96. Jones, D. M., C. Squires and K. Roduhl. "Effect of rope skipping on physical work capacity." Research Quarterly. 33:236, 1962.

97. Karlsson, J. "Lactate and phosphagan concentrations in working muscle of man." Acta Physiological Scandinavica. (supplement), 358:1-72, 1974.

98. Karvonen, M., K. Kentala and O. Muslala. "The effects of training heart rate: a longitudinal study." Ann. Med. Exptl. Biol. Fenn. 35:307-315, 1957.

99. Katch, F. K. and W. D. McArdle. Nutrition, Weight Control, and Exercise. Boston: Houghton Mifflin Company, 1977.

100. Keelor, R. O., Address to 1976 Blue Shield Annual Program Conference, President's Council on Physical Fitness and Sports, 1976.

101. Keynotes. 9:1, 1979, National Industrial Recreation Association, Chicago.

102. Klein, K. K. and J. C. Buckley. "Asymmetries of growth of the pelvis and legs of growing children." Unpublished study, 1967.

103. Kraus, H. Principles and Practices of Therapeutic Exercise. Springfield, Ill: Charles. C. Thomas, Publisher, 1949.

104. Lamb, D. R. Physiology of Exercise Responses and Adaptations. New York: Macmillian Publishing Company, Inc., 1978.

105. Link, M. M. Space Medicine in Project Mercury. NASA SP-4003, 1965.

106. Maas, S. H. "A study of the cardiovascular training effects of aerobic dance instruction among college age females." Master's Thesis. North Texas State University, 1975.

107. Manzer, C. W. "An experimental investigation of rest pauses." Archives of Psychology. 90:76, 1947.

108. Mathews, D. K. and E. L. Fox. <u>The Physiological Basis of Physical Education and Athletics</u>. Philadelphia, PA: W. B. Saunders Company, 1976.

109. Mathews, D. K. and R. Kruse. "Effect of isometric and isotonic exercise on elbow flexor muscle groups." <u>Research Quarterly</u>. 28:26-37, 1957.

110. Mayer, J. <u>Overweight</u>. Englewood Cliffs, N.J: Prentice-Hall, 1968.

111. McArdle, W. D., J. R. Magel and L. C. Kyvallos. "Aerobic capacity, heart rate and estimated energy cost during women's competitive basketball." <u>Research Quarterly</u>. 42:178-186, 1972.

112. Meyers, C. R. "Effects of two isometric routines on strength, size and endurance in exercised and non-exercised arms." <u>Research Quarterly</u>. 38:430-440, 1967.

113. Mole, P., L. Oscai and J. Holloszy. "Adaptation of muscle to exercise. Increase in levels of palmityl CoA synthease, carnitine palmityltransferase and palmityl CoA dehydrogenase, and in the capacity to oxidize fats." <u>Journal of Clinical Investigation</u>. 50:2323-2330, 1971.

114. Morgan, T. L., Cobb, F. Short, R. Ross and D. Gunn. "Effects of long term exercise on human muscle mitachondria." <u>Muscle Metabolism During Exercise</u>. Pernow, B. and New York: Plenum Press, 1971.

115. Muller, E. A. and W. Rohmert. "Die geschwindigkeit der muskeldraft zunahme bei isometrischen training." <u>Arbeitsphysiologie</u>. 19:403-419, 1963.

116. Nadel, J. A. and J. H. Comroe, Jr. "Acute effects of inhalation of cigarette smoke on airway conduction." <u>Journal of Applied Physiology</u>. 16:713-716, 1961.

117. Nisbett, R. E. "Eating behavior and obesity in men and animals." <u>Advances in Psychosomatic Medicine</u>. 7:173-193, 1972.

118. Nygaard, E. and E. Nielsen. "Skeletal muscle fiber capillarization with extreme endurance training in man." <u>Swimming Medicine IV</u>. International Series on Sport Sciences. Ed. B. Eriksson and B. Furberg, University Park Press, Baltimore, Md, 1978.

119. Oscai, L. B., S. P. Babirak, F. B. Dubach, J. M. McGarr and C. N. Spirakis, "Exercise or food restriction: effect on adipose tissue cellularity." <u>American Journal of Physiology</u>. 27:901-904, 1974.

120. Paffenberger, R. S., Jr., and W. E. Hale. "Work activity and coronary heart mortality." <u>New England Journal of Medicine</u>, 292(11):545-50, 1975.

121. Parr, R. B. and J. H. Wilmore, "Professional basketball players: athletic profiles." <u>The Physician and Sports Medicine</u>, 6:106-110, 1978.

122. Pipes, T. V. and J. H. Wilmore, "Isokinetic vs isotonic strength training in adult men." <u>Medicine and Science in Sports</u>.

123. Pipes, T. V. "Variable resistance vs constant resistance strength training in adult males." <u>European Journal of Applied Physiology</u>. 39:27-35, 1978.

124. Pollock, M. L., G. A. Dawson H. S. Miller, A. Ward, D. Cooper, W. Headley, A. C. Linnerud and A. Nomeir. "Physiological responses of men 49 to 65 years of age to endurance training." Journal of American Geriatrics Society. 24:97-104, 1976.

125. Pollock, M. L., H. Miller, R. Janeway, A. C. Linnerud, B. Robertson and R. Valentino. "Effects of walking on body composition and cardiovascular function in middle-aged men." Journal of Applied Physiology. 30:126-130, 1971.

126. Pollock, M. L., H. S. Miller, Jr., A. C. Linnerud, C. L. Royster, W. E. Smith and W. H. Sonner. "Physiological findings in well-trained middle-aged American men." British Association of Sports Medicine Journal. 7: 222-229, 1973.

127. Pollock, M. L., J. Ayres, A. Ward, J. Sass and S. White. "Working capacity, cardiorespiratory, and body composition characteristics of world class middle and long distance runners." The Physiologist. 18:355, 1975.

128. Pollock, M. L., J. H. Wilmore and S. E. Fox III. Health and Fitness Through Physical Activity. New York: John Wiley and Sons, 1978.

129. Pollock, M. L., L. Gettman, A. Jackson, J. Ayres, A. Ward and A. C. Linnerud. "Body composition of elite class distance runners." Annals of the New York Academy of Sciences. 301:361-370, 1977.

130. Pollock, M. L., L. R. Gettman, C. A. Milesis, M. D. Bah, L. Durstine and R. B. Johnson. "Effects of frequency and duration of training on attrition and incidence of injury." Medicine and Science in Sports. 9:31-36, 1977.

131. Pollock, M. L. "Physiological characteristics of champion track athletes. Track and Field Quarterly. 74:215-221, 1974.

132. Pollock, M. L. "Physiological characteristics of older champion track athletes." Research Quarterly. 45:363-373, 1976.

133. Pollock, M. L. "The effects of walking on body composition and cardiovascular function of middle-aged men." Journal of Applied Physiology. 30:126, 1974.

134. Pollock, M. L. "The quantification of endurance training programs." In Exercise and Sport Sciences Reviews. Vol 1. J. H. Wilmore (ed). New York: Academic Press, 1973.

135. Pravosudov, V. "The effects of physical exercise on health and economic efficiency Lesgaft State Institute of Physical Culture-Leningrad, USSR, 1975.

136. Rasch, P. J. "Progressive resistance exercise: isotonic and isometric: a review. Journal of the Association for Physical and Mental Rehabilitation. 15:46-50, 56, 1961.

137. Rarick, G. L. and G. L. Larson. "Observation on frequency and intensity of isometric muscular effort in developing static strength in post-pubescent males." Research Quarterly. 29:333-341, 1958.

138. Raven, P. B., L. R. Gettman, M. L. Pollock and K. H. Cooper. "A physiological evaluation of professional soccer players." Brit**ish Journal of Sports Medicine**. 10:209-216, 1976.

139. Rummel, J. A., C. F. Sawin, E. L. Michel, M. C. Buderer and W. T. Thornton. "Exericse and long duration space flight through 84 days." Journal of the American Women's Association. 30:173-187, 1975.

140. Saltin, B. G. Blomquist, G. Mitchel, R. L. Johnson, J. K. Wildenthal and C. B. Chapman. "Response to exercise after bed rest and training. A longitudinal study of adaptative changes on oxygen transport and body composition." Circulation, 38:1-78, 1968.

141. Sawin, C. F. and J. A. Rummel and E. L. Michel. "Instrumental personal exercise during long-duration space flights." Avaiation Space and Environmental Medicine, 46:394-400, 1975.

142. Schanche, D. A. "Diet books that can poison your mind and harm your body." Today's Health. :56-61, 1974.

143. Sheehan, G. A. Medical Advice for Runners. Mountain View, CA: World Publications 1978.

144. Stamford, B. A., A. Weltman, R. H. Moffatt and C. Fulco. "Status of police officers with regard to select. cardiorespiratory and body composition and fitness variables." Medicine and Science in Sports. 10:294-297, 1978.

145. Subotnick, S. I. Common Cures for Running Injuries. Mountain View, CA: World Publications, 1979.

146. Subotnick, S. I. The Running Foot Doctor. Mountain View, CA: World Publications, 1977.

147. Syster, B. and G. Stull. "Muscular endurance retention as a function of the length of detraining." Research Quarterly. 41:105-109, 1970.

148. Thorstensson, A. L. Larson, P. Tesch and J. Karlsson. "Muscle strength and fiber type composition in athletes and sedentary men." Medicine and Science in Sports. 9:26-30, 1977.

149. Ullyot, J. Women's Running. Mountain View, CA: World Publications, 1976.

150. Vail, S. S. "Changes in the muscles of the limbs in overtraining, in trained and untrained animals." Arkhiv Patologii (Russian). 29:45-49, 1967.

151. Van Pelt, W. L., S. Meyers and J. Holland. "1978 Houston Marathon: lower extremity injuries and running shoes." Personal Communication. 1978.

152. Waldman, R. and G. Stull. "Effect of various periods of inactivity on retention of newly acquired levels of muscular endurance." Research Quarterly. 40:396-401, 1969.

153. Weber, H. "The energy cost of aerobic dancing." Fitness for Living. 8:26, 1974.

154. Wells, K. F. Kinesiology. Philadelpha: W. B. Saunders, Company, 1971.

155. Wilmore, J. "Alterations in strength, body composition and anthropometric measurements consequent to a 10-week weight training program." Medicine and Science in Sports. 6:133-138, 1974.

156. Wilmore, J. H. Athletic Training and Physical Fitness. Boston: Allyn and Bacon, Inc. 1976.

157. Wilmore, J. H. and W. L. Haskell. "Body composition and endurance capacity of professional football players." Journal of Applied Physiology, 33:564-567, 1972.

158. Wilmore, J. H., H. L. Miller and M. L. Pollock. "Body Composition and physiological characteristics of active endurance athletes in their eighth decade of life." Medicine and Science in Sports. 6:44-48, 1974.

159. Wilmore, J. H. "Letter to the editor." Medicine and Science in Sports. 11: , 1979

160. Wilmore, J. H., R. B. Parr, P. Ward, P. A. Vodak, T. J. Barstow, T. V. Pipes, G. Grimditch and P. Leslie. "Energy cost of circuit weight training." Medicine and Science in Sports. 10:75-78, 1978.

161. Wilmore, J. H., R. B. Parr, R. N. Girandola, P. Ward, P. A. Vodak, T. J. Barstow, T. V. Pipes, G. T. Romero and P. Leslie. "Physiological alterations consequent to circuit weight training." Medicine and Science in Sports. 10:79-84, 1978.

162. Wilson, T. B., R. Wanzel, V. Gillespie and C. J. Robers. An introduction to Industrial Recreation. Dubuque, Iowa: Wm. C. Brown Company Publishers, 1979.

163. Wyndom, C. H. and N. B. Strydom. "The danger of inadequate water intake during marathon running." South African Medical Journal. 43:893-896, 1969.

CPSIA information can be obtained at www.ICGtesting.com
Printed in the USA
LVOW09s0243040216

473641LV00013B/135/P